SANTA CRUZ CITY-COUNTY LIBRARY SYSTEM

0000115899148

D0605686

ACU
2482

810.8035 Healer.
HEA

DATE			

DISCARDED

SANTA CRUZ PUBLIC LIBRARY
Santa Cruz, California

BAKER & TAYLOR

ARCHETYPES OF THE COLLECTIVE UNCONSCIOUS
VOLUME 2
Reflecting American Culture Through Literature and Art

HEALER

TRANSFORMING THE INNER AND OUTER WOUNDS

Introduction by Andrew Weil

JEREMY P. TARCHER/PUTNAM
A MEMBER OF PENGUIN PUTNAM INC.
NEW YORK

A BOOK LABORATORY BOOK

Most Tarcher/Putnam books are available at special quantity discounts for bulk purchase for sales promotions, premiums, fund-raising, and educational needs. Special books or book excerpts also can be created to fit specific needs. For details, write Putnam Special Markets, 375 Hudson Street, New York, NY 10014.

Jeremy P. Tarcher/Putnam
A member of
Penguin Putnam Inc.
375 Hudson Street
New York, NY 10014
www.penguinputnam.com
Introduction © Robert A. Johnson
Searching for Love Through Stories and Art © Mark Robert Waldman
Designed by Kristen Garneau, Garneau Design, Sausalito, CA

All rights reserved. This book, or parts thereof, may not be reproduced in any form without permission. Published simultaneously in Canada.

Library of Congress Cataloging-in-Publications Data

Healer: dancing with the healing spirit / introduction by Andrew Weil.
        p. cm.—(Archetypes of the collective unconscious ; v. 2)
     "A Book Laboratory book"—T.p. verso
  ISBN 1-58542-188-X
    1. Medicine—Literary collections. 2. Healers—Literary collections. 3. Healing—Literary collections. 4. Health—Literary collections. 5. American Literature. I. Series.
  PS648.M36H43 2002   2002028701
810.8'0356—dc21

Printed in Singapore
10 9 8 7 6 5 4 3 2 1

TABLE OF CONTENTS

ABOUT   THIS   SERIES

OUR WORLD IS FILLED WITH ARCHETYPAL IMAGERY, POWERFUL SYMBOLS THAT REFLECT THE DEEPEST LAYERS OF OUR personality—our strengths, weaknesses, and unacknowledged gifts that lay hidden within our souls. Primarily unconscious, these inner forces shape our behaviors, attitudes and beliefs. By exploring these secret desires—in ourselves, through literature and art—we can gain mastery over them, bringing greater consciousness into our lives.

Archetypal themes are universal, for they can be found in every culture throughout history. But each society reflects them in distinctive ways. The American lover, for example, is far more romantic, erotic, and idealized than the images portrayed in Asia. By contrast, the Shadow, which is aptly acknowledged in the European psyche, is relatively ignored by Americans. Unlike other cultures, we do not like to peer directly at the darkness that lies within. Instead we project our shadows onto fiction, the movies, or the criminal elements in the world. Even the shadow artists in America are often met with hostility or disdain, especially when the subject offends our moral and religious values. The shadow artist is readily condemned, an unpatriotic pariah that spoils our fantasies and dreams.

The American seeker is also unique amongst the cultures of the world: in our separation of church from state, religion becomes a quest for personal spirituality, one that liberally borrows from other traditions and groups. Our economic and scientific advancements have also transformed the healer archetype from a country shaman into a medical sage.

Artists, poets, and writers help to bring these archetypal forms to life by embracing them in their work. Stephen King, for example, is a master of the shadow, as was Sexton, Poe, and Melville. The spiritual quest of the seeker is vividly captured in the poetry of Whitman and Frost, in the prose of Alice Walker, and in the speeches of Martin Luther King. Even the face of Andrew Weil, alternative medicine's champion, has become a core archetypal symbol of the American healer: wise, warm, and passionately devoted to the integration of body, mind, and soul. And who would not be moved by O'Henry's *The Gift of the Magi* in which two lovers sacrifice their most valued possessions to soothe each other's heart?

Art in particular makes a strong impression upon our soul, and in choosing the illustrations to accompany these stories, we have selected unique images that span the breadth and depth of contemporary American painting and photography. From the sun-dappled colors of the impressionists, to the austere contrasts of black and white photography, and from the immediacy of the advertising medium and the obliqueness of the symbolic form, these images hint at the acuity of our inner landscapes and dreams. Mysterious, moody, and serene, they work upon our psyches inviting us to rest the eye upon the symbolic eloquence of life.

May these stories and images guide you inwards as you will witness that wondrous place where a greater consciousness resides.

The wonder of the collective unconscious is that it is all there, all the legend and history of the human race, with its unexorcised demons and its gentle saints, its mysteries and its wisdom, all with each one of us—a microcosm with the macrocosm. The exploration of this world is more challenging than the exploration of the solar system; and the journey to inner space is not necessarily an easy or a safe trip.

—June Singer

The archetype represents a profound riddle surpassing our rational comprehension [expressing] itself first and foremost in metaphors. There is some part of its meaning that always remains unknown and defies formulation.

—Jacobi Jolande

Our personal psychology is just a thin skin, a ripple on the ocean of collective psychology [and] the archetypes are the great decisive forces, they bring about the real events, and not our personal reasoning and practical intellect . . . . The archetypal images decide the fate of man.

—Carl G. Jung

Series Editor: Mark Robert Waldman
Series conceived by Jeremy P. Tarcher
Series created by Philip Dunn, Manuela Dunn Mascetti and Book Laboratory
Picture research by Julie Foakes
Design by Kristen Garneau

Other Titles in the Series:
Shadow: Touching the Darkness Within, Volume 1, with an Introduction by Robert Bly
Seeker: Traveling the Path to Enlightenment, Volume 3, with an Introduction by Jean Houston
Lover: Embracing Our Passionate Hearts, Volume 4, with an Introduction by Robert A. Johnson

THE   HEALER   ARCHETYPE

by Andrew Weil

WHEN PEOPLE ARE SICK, INJURED, AND IN PAIN, THEY OFTEN IMAGINE MAGICAL, INSTANTANEOUS CURES. IN THEIR fantasies external agents or agencies are usually central: the healer god Apollo, for example, or Jesus or the Virgin Mary, a Hindu saint, a sacred grotto, a marvelous fountain, or a rare stone. Interaction with such a being or thing takes away suffering, comforts, brings ease, and restores wholeness. Restoration of wholeness is the literal meaning of healing.

A Freudian might argue that these fantasies derive from one's earliest experiences of infancy in which mother is the ultimate source of comfort. An infant's cry usually brings quick relief from whatever is wrong through the agency of an all-powerful being who temporarily re-establishes the security and wholeness of life in the womb. Whatever its psychological origins, the belief that healing comes from outside is deep-seated and powerful, often persisting throughout life.

As a physician who practices and teaches integrative medicine with an emphasis on natural healing, I am aware that I am a focus for the projections of the hopes and fears of patients, many of whom would have me play the role of healer. I am also well aware that belief is a powerful influence on the outcome of treatment. As a scientist I am fascinated by the potential for healing that all living organisms share, and my experiences in medicine, both as a doctor and as a patient, convince me that the true source of healing is inside us, not outside. Knowing this, and also knowing that most patients want me to heal them, creates a complex dynamic, one that must be managed skillfully and delicately. What is called for is medicine as art, not as science.

My contention that healing is innate is hardly an original idea. Hippocrates articulated it in the fifth century, B.C., when he admonished physicians to revere the healing power of nature (the *vis medicatrix naturae*). Since his time, thoughtful medical philosophers in disparate cultures have developed their theories and systems from the same premise: that healing comes from within and must be stimulated, activated, or unblocked by therapeutic action to allow it to express itself. Healing comes from within, treatment from without; at best, treatment facilitates healing. In modern Western culture this idea has been lost in our enthusiasm for medical technology, especially powerful drugs and invasive procedures that reinforce the illusion of external causation. An example I often use in teaching medical students is a case of a patient critically ill with bacterial pneumonia. The patient is hospitalized, given intravenous antibiotics, and within hours is out of danger. What happened? It certainly looks as if the antibiotics caused the cure. But a more precise analysis shows that the antibiotics knocked down populations of invading bacteria down to levels where the patient's immune system was able to take over and finish the job, a task it was unable to do because it was overwhelmed. That is, the treatment facilitated innate mechanisms of defense and regeneration that restored the balance of health. One of the most succinct expressions of this process I ever read was the motto of a medical club I belonged to: "We dress the wound, God heals it." (Of course, I understand "God" here to mean Nature in its wondrous, mysterious, and beneficent aspect.) What then of human healers? I have met and worked with extraordinary practitioners with impressive track records of clinical success. Some were conventional physicians, some unconventional, and some were laypersons without any professional training or credentials. Some of them were clearly skilled at facilitating healing. For example, Robert Fulford, an old osteopathic physician I have described elsewhere was a master of manual medicine— gentle, hands-on manipulation of the physical structure of the body. He routinely cured children of recurrent ear infections with this method, saying that his adjustments in the musculoskeletal system simply allowed "old Mother Nature to do her job."

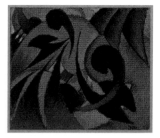

Above: Arthur Dove, *Nature Symbolized No. 2.*

Another healer I have worked with, Rosalyn Bruyere, reads patients' energy fields to diagnose problems and channels energy through her hands to relieve them. I have felt this energy and have experienced it as anything but subtle, even though I do not know how to explain it in scientific terms. And I have seen cures follow her treatments. Still, my interpretation is that they result from facilitation or activation or unblocking of innate healing, even if by means unfamiliar to medical scientists. Furthermore, I know that belief in treatments and practitioners greatly contributes to the outcomes.

The practice of healing lies in the heart. If your heart is false, the physician within you will be false.

—Paracelsus

Years ago at Columbia University, I took a memorable course in medical hypnosis that strongly influenced my thinking about mind/body interactions. I learned first that trance is a natural, innate capacity of human beings that varies in degree from person to person. I learned also that a hypnotist does not really do anything to a subject, but simply arranges circumstances to increase the probability of a subject shifting into an altered state of awareness that helps to focus attention and increase suggestibility. A key factor in this interaction is the subject's expectation of being hypnotized. And as hypnotists get better through practice, it becomes ever easier for them to hypnotize, because their reputations precede them—that is, they produce greater expectations of being hypnotized. In hypnosis circles this "power" is called the "aura" of the hypnotist—his or her potential to create in the subject the expectation of being hypnotized. In the same way powerful healers create expectation of being healed. That belief enhances their treatments and through the many possible avenues of mind/body communication helps activate innate mechanisms of healing. Skilled practitioners know how to work with expectation creatively. They can take the projected beliefs of patients and reflect them back in ways that increase the probability of healing responses.

In the 1970s I lived and worked in Colombia, Ecuador, and Peru, studying medicinal plants and shamanism. I was much interested in supernatural, magical healing. Although I did find magic in the shamanic world I visited, it was not supernatural. It was the same magic that goes on in the offices of doctors and therapists on much more familiar ground: the projection and reflection of belief and its translation into physiological responses that may interact productively with externally applied treatments to activate and direct the healing power of nature. The most effective shamans I met were master psychotherapists who understood intuitively the belief systems of clients and knew how to impact them in the service of healing.

There is something of the Wizard of Oz in the healer archetype. The great and powerful Oz turned out to be a very ordinary man with no extraordinary powers at all, but by working with the projected beliefs of Dorothy and her friends, he was able to inspire them to draw on their own resources to overcome all obstacles. And the charade was necessary. Without the smoke and mirrors, the desired outcome might not have occurred.

This is exactly the paradox of the healer archetype and the demand it places on all who wish to identify with it to practice with great sensitivity and skill. Healing is not the physician's gift to bestow.

All a good doctor or therapist can do is arrange circumstances to increase the probability of healing. But part of that arranging of circumstances might include playing the expected role of the giver of healing. One might ask why it is that we cannot simply will healing in ourselves without projecting belief onto external agents and agencies. If the mind can truly interact with the body, why can't it do the necessary activating or unblocking of the mechanisms of the body's healing system? The answer to that question must have to do with the nature of will and its relationship to the physical underpinnings of consciousness. I often say that the part of the mind where will is located is not the part that connects directly to the nervous system and the controls of our physiology. One day we might understand that statement more precisely in neuropsychiatric terms, we will still be left with the practical problem: in order to influence those controls, most of us have to project belief onto something external, then interact with that person or thing. I say "most of us" because it appears that some people, through psychospiritual practice or inborn talent, can directly influence the functions of the body others only experience as "involuntary."

What practical advice follows from this view of healing and healers? I would caution patients to choose their healers carefully. There is an element of authoritarianism in the doctor-patient relationship, an inequality of power that may be unavoidable if the magic of the healer is to occur. If you are going to turn over your power to an external authority, be sure it is someone whose ethics are impeccable.

I would urge practitioners to ponder the complexities of their relationships with patients and try to find a middle way through the opposing pulls they will feel, lest we identify too strongly with the healer archetype and lose sight of the true source of healing, or reject it in a desire to be an equal partner with the patient and lose the ability to facilitate healing maximally. This requires constant vigilance.

In the following essays, you will find many of these themes. Ram Dass, in writing about his stroke, describes his healing in terms of adaptation to loss. He cannot walk, his speech is impaired, but he fully accepts these changes and remains an effective teacher. In Lewis Thomas's affectionate portrait of his physician father you will feel the discomfort of one doctor with the healer archetype. The elder Thomas has developed an aura of healer that he feels is undeserved. Eventually he quits medicine for the practice of surgery, where he feels he can do "real" treatment. And Anatole Broyard's tale of trying to find the right urologist underscores the importance of right chemistry between patient and practitioner.

If the healer only seems to cause healing, a good practitioner of the healing art can nonetheless bring needed knowledge, enthusiasm, and attention to the medical encounter. I often see references to "the wounded healer," suggesting that suffering is required to play the role well, it is true that a physician who has experienced illness or injury is more likely to empathize with a patient. In any case, if the interaction between healer and patient succeeds, both parties learn from the experience. Both are changed by it and grow from it.

T R A N S F O R M I N G   O U R   W O U N D S
T H R O U G H   S T O R I E S   A N D   A R T

by Mark Robert Waldman, Series Editor

> *In a sense, medicine is burning, as old ideas and methods are fading on every hand. But medicine's fires are purifying; new life is emerging from the ashes, as it always does . . . and healing is in the wind. The rebirth has begun.*
>
> —Larry Dossey, Former Panel Chair, *National Institutes of Health*

Throughout history, the image of the healer has radiated a mystical light, guiding us through our inner and outer wounds. We have seen the healer as both charlatan and sage—a dispenser of snake oil, a purveyor of herbs, the preacher who nurtures our soul—but for most Americans, the cardinal symbols of the healer have been the doctor, psychiatrist and nurse. These are the people to whom we entrust ourselves when illness or injury strikes. The healer of today no longer comes to our homes, as did the doctor of yesteryear; nor does he mend our souls. Instead, he has become a specialist of the body: we travel to medical suites equipped with technological wizardry, and we wander the aisles of drugstores, lost in a pharmacological maze. Our healing capacities have phenomenally grown, but in the process we may have sacrificed something essential, even sacred. As Frederick Stenn, Associate Professor at Northwestern Medical School, laments:

> *Most physicians have lost the pearl that was once an intimate part of the medicine, and that is humanism. Machinery, efficiency and precision have driven from the heart warmth, compassion, sympathy, and concern for the individual. Medicine is now an icy science; its charm belongs to another age.*

In response to the sterility now felt, a new generation of healers has emerged, reinvesting our science with warmth. Our interest in alternative medicine has soared as practitioners continue to employ unusual treatments gathered from indigenous cultures abroad. Supported by university research and government grants, our weapons for healing include acupuncture, herbology, meditation, biofeedback, and life-style enhancement. Even the power of prayer is being investigated, harboring a growing philosophy of health that integrates body, spirit, and mind. For example, in the treatment of heart disease and cancer, doctors routinely use stress reduction techniques (breathing, yoga, relaxation, guided imagery, etc.) in conjunction with psychotherapy, discussion groups, and dietary advice. To recover from illness, we are asked to reevaluate our work habits and to invest ourselves in social pursuits. We are even challenged to reappraise our fears about aging and death.

This new approach to healing is changing the way we think about disease. Led by respected physicians and researchers like Bernie Siegal, Oliver Sacks, Larry Dossey, Deepak Chopra, Herbert Benson, Dean Ornish and others, we have begun to shift our focus towards a holistic view, one in which the doctor and patient are seen as equal partners in one's pursuit of health. These new healers are moving away from their positions of authority, acting instead as compassionate educators and guides.

The tales and memoirs in this anthology explore these evolving themes, depicting the image of an uncertain healer who must stand guardian over our inner and outer worlds. Where does the power really lie, asks William Carlos Williams in his story, *The Use of Force:* in the doctor or the patient, in the illness or one's health? Williams, like other authors in this volume, was a physician who reached deeply into his unconscious to construct his literary themes.

We are returning, as a collective awareness, to the understanding that the body is in fact not separate from the mind . . . Thoughts of aggression, unforgiveness, conflict and fear, tear down the body because they tear down the soul. Healed thoughts produce healing, in body as well as mind.

—Marianne Williamson

Writers often use their illnesses to expose the dilemmas that patients often face: Will my doctor understand, will she listen to my fears? In the essay by Oliver Sacks, he asks the following question: "Is my patient's problem a virus or a gift, and should it be savored or cured?" And what if the patient dies? Does this mean that the doctor has failed? And if traditional medicine offers no cure, what alternatives remain? The memoirs of Caroline Myss and Donna Eden explore the intuitive and energetic realms of healing.

The way in which we grapple with mortality and disease plays a significant role in our lives, and these themes, too, are reflected in this book. "Can I love my cancerous disease?" ponders Marjorie Gross. Other authors raise similar issues: "Am I capable of accepting all the parts of myself: my nose, my fat, my slowly encroaching death?" If we do not confront these issues, we may deprive ourselves of meaningful insights about life.

And what can our art illuminate about the archetypal healer in America?

The archetypal energy of healer can reach beyond the individual to address the ills of society as well. But who will these leaders be? Who will nurture our wounded world, and who will guide us towards healing the hunger of the poor, the disenfranchised, the victims of future wars? Will we be able to discern the difference between those who genuinely care and those who simply seek power over others? The healer, like every archetypal force, has its shadow side: the surgeon can turn greedy or careless, the patient can simmer with blame, the healer can even kill. In future generations, questions concerning mortality, euthanasia, overpopulation, and the right to life will urge us to rethink our definitions of health, which raises yet another difficult question: Who ultimately has control over our bodies and our lives: our selves, our families, the government, or the church? Only when we have the courage to look within, to muster our compassion and love in the face of illness and disease, will our healing powers shine. As Carl Jung once wrote, the healer's knowledge is "like a flickering lamp, the one dim light in the darkness." Medicine is burning, and healing is in the wind.

Right: Marsden Hartley, *Movements.*

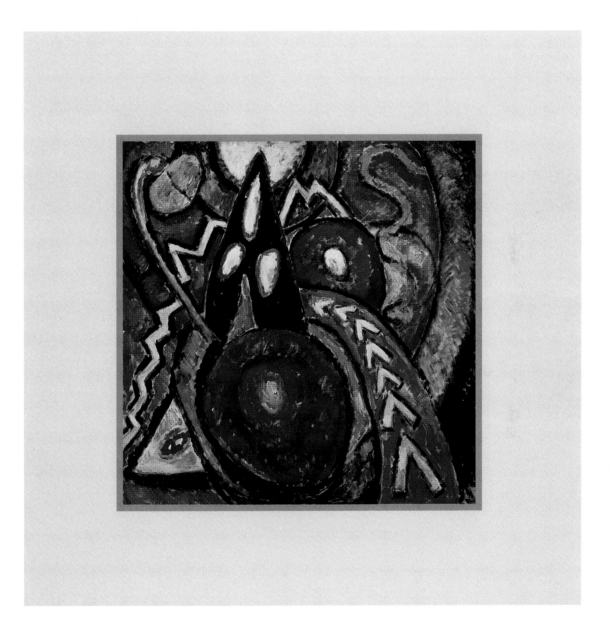

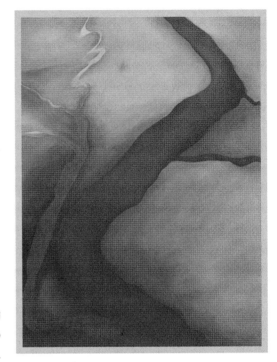

HEART ATTACK

Max Apple

MY SICKNESS BOTHERS ME, THOUGH I PERSIST IN denying it. It is indigestion I think and eat no onions; gout and I order no liver or goose. The possibility of nervous exhaustion keeps me abed for three days, breathing deeply. I do yoga for anxiety. But, finally, here I am amid magazines awaiting, naked to the waist, cough at the balls, needle in the vein. From my viral pneumonia days, I remember his Sheaffers desk set and the 14kt. gold point. It writes prescriptions without a scratch. In the time of the bad sunburn, my damaged eyes scanned the walls reading degrees and being jealous of the good-looking woman, the three boys, the weeping willow in the back yard.

I have a choice of *Sports Illustrated*, *Time*, *Boy's World*, others. As if by design, I choose the free pamphlet on the wall. Fleischmann's Margarine gives me some straight talk about cholesterol. I remember the ten thousand eggs of my youth, those miracles of protein that have perhaps made my interior an artgum eraser. Two over easy in the morning, a hard one every night, poached, sometimes eviscerated by mayonnaise. In many ways I have been an egg man. The pamphlet shows my heart, a small pump the size of my fist. I make a fist and stare at knuckles, white as the eggshells I wish I had eaten instead. Where did I learn that your penis is the size of your middle finger plus the distance that finger can reach down your arm. Mine cannot make it to the wrist. My heart too must be a pea in this flimsy, hairless chest.

Above: Georgia O'Keeffe, *It Was Yellow and Pink IIII.*

From a door marked PRIVATE a nurse, all in white, comes to me. She sits very close on the couch and looks down at my pamphlet. She takes my damp hand in hers and tickles my palm. Her soft lips against my ear whisper musically, "Every cloud has a silver lining . . . ."

"But arteries," I respond, "my arteries are caked with the mistakes of my youth."

She points to the pamphlet. "Arteries should be lined only with their moist little selves. Be good to your arteries, be kind to your heart. It's the only one you'll ever have." She puts her tongue in my ear, and one arm reaches under my shirt. She sings, "A fella needs a girl . . . ."

"I need a doctor . . . my arteries."

She points again to the pamphlet and reads, "Arteries, though similar to, are more important than girls in several ways. Look at this one pink and flexible as a Speidel band. Over there threatens cholesterol, dark as motor oil, thick as birthday cake. Cholesterol is the bully of the body. It picks on blood, good honest blood who bothers no one and goes happily between the races, creeds, and colors."

"I have pains," I tell her, "pains in my chest and my tongue feels fat and moss grows in my joints."

She unbuttons my shirt slowly. Her long cool fingers cup me as if I were all breasts. Her clever right hand is at my back counting vertebrae. She takes off the stiff nurse's cap and nuzzles my solar plexus. Into my middle she hums, "I'm as corny as Kansas in August . . ." The vibrations go deep. She responds to me. "There," I gasp, "right there." I am overcome as if by Valium. As I moan she moves me down on the cracking vinyl couch. Her lips, teeth, and tongue fire between my ribs. She hums Muzak and the room spins until I sight the pamphlet clinging to a bobby pin. In my ecstasy, I see the diagram of cholesterol, in peaks and valleys, nipping at blood that makes its way, like a hero, through the narrow places.

When she lets me up, I am bruised but feeling wonderful. Her lips are colorless from the pressure she has exerted upon me. I start to take off my trousers. She stays my hand at the belt buckle, kisses me long. "The oath," she whispers.

"I'm cured," I say. "Forget him. Forget the urine and the blood. Look." I beat my chest like Tarzan, I spit across the room into a tiny bronze ashtray.

"I'll pack," she says. She goes into PRIVATE while I pick out a few *Reader's Digests* for the road, *Today's Health* for the bathroom. She returns carrying a centrifuge and a rack of test tubes. We embrace, then I bend to help with her things.

"Don't be cruel," she whispers, "to a heart that's true. . ."

On the way out we throw a kiss to the pharmacist and my blood slips through.

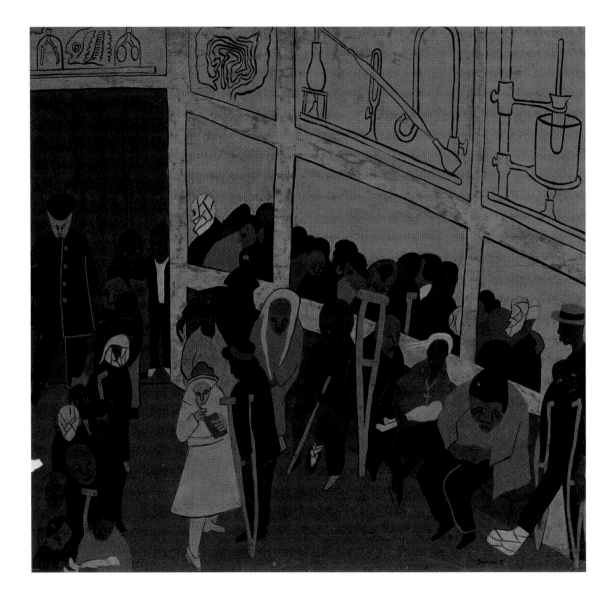

HEALING AND THE MIND

Bill Moyers

S IRENS WAIL THROUGH THE NIGHT AS AMBULANCE AFTER AMBULANCE PULLS UP TO THE EMERGENCY ROOM OF PARKLAND Memorial Hospital, the public hospital in Dallas, Texas. The emergency area is so crowded that patients' beds line the hallways. Anyone who does not need immediate medical attention is sent to a packed waiting area. Men, women, and children sit silently, often in pain, waiting for hours to see a doctor. During the day more than 350 people may cram the waiting area of the outpatient clinic, until the line extends beyond the hospital door to the sidewalk. It is not unusual for some of these people, most of them poor, to wait ten or twelve hours to receive fifteen minutes of basic medical care. Like all public hospitals, Parkland is underfunded, overcrowded, and overwhelmed. Yet unlike most, it has resolved to change the way it practices medicine.

The man behind the change is Dr. Ron Anderson, Parkland's chief executive officer, a practicing internist and a Southern Baptist who has been influenced both by Native American wisdom about healing and by clinical experience demonstrating that patients benefit measurably when their medical treatment includes attention to their emotional needs.

Following Ron Anderson on his rounds with medical students, I listen as he stops at the bedside of an

Left: Jacob Lawrence, *Free Clinic.*

elderly woman suffering from chronic asthma. He asks the usual questions: "How did you sleep last night?" "Is the breathing getting any easier?" His next questions surprise the medical students: "Is your son looking for work?" "Is he still drinking?" "Tell us what happened right before the asthma attack." He explains to his puzzled students, "We know that anxiety aggravates many illnesses, especially chronic conditions like asthma. So we have to find out what may be causing her episodes of stress and help her find some way of coping with it. Otherwise, she will land in here again, and next time we might not be able to save her. We cannot just prescribe medication and walk away. That is medical neglect. We have to take the time to get to know her, how she lives, her values, what her social supports are. If we don't know that her son is her sole support and that he's out of work, we will be much less effective in dealing with her asthma."

Modern medicine, with all its extraordinary technology, has accomplished wonders, but Anderson believes that caring is also a powerful medicine. The most striking example of his emphasis can be seen in Parkland's neonatal intensive care unit. Like hospitals across the country, Parkland is dealing with a sharp increase in premature and low-birth-weight babies. The hospital employs the latest technology to keep those infants alive, but saving them, Anderson says, is not enough. Equally important is promoting the emotional connection between parent and child. Scientific research has shown that without human contact, a baby will wither and its normal development will be stunted. Babies need to be touched.

Cindy Wheeler is a neonatal nurse. I watch as she introduces Vanessa, a fifteen year-old mother, to her premature son for the first time. In a room outside the intensive care unit, Vanessa scrubs her hands and arms. Cindy helps her put a sterilized gown over her clothing and then don a mask that covers her nose and mouth. They proceed through the double doors into a series of open rooms with row after row of high-tech medical machinery. In the middle of these islands of hardware is an incubator, a technological womb for Malcolm, Vanessa's tiny son. Protected by this space-age bubble, Malcolm looks more like a fetus than a baby. He is covered with tape and dotted with intravenous needles; tubes connect him to a series of monitors and machines. Cindy knows that Vanessa is frightened and wants to run away. She takes the mother's hand and in a gentle voice begins to tell her that it will be okay, that the baby needs her. She guides Vanessa's finger to Malcolm's miniature hand, whispering that all babies, no matter how old, will respond to the touch of a mother's hand by gripping her finger. The moment is crucial. Vanessa's tense ambivalence will either disappear or cause her to flee. The tiny hand closes around her middle finger. The mother smiles and closes her eyes. Her relief is palpable.

For many women like Vanessa, Cindy tells me, a baby is a status symbol, the first they can call their own. Their dream of a Gerber baby, a Barbie doll, is shattered when the child is born very small or critically ill. "Our mission," she says, "is to share our understanding of the loss they feel, and to help the mothers feel something positive from what otherwise can be a major disappointment and leave a deep psychological scar."

Many of the young mothers are from dysfunctional families. The hospital staff is often the closest they have come to having a nurturing family, and their experience in the neonatal unit is for some the first time they feel supported. To Cindy Wheeler and her colleagues, these teenage mothers are forced to make a decisive choice: to continue being controlled by their problems, or to take charge of their circumstances and, through caring, to make a difference. "Sometimes," says Cindy, "we get very angry at the mothers. A while ago, we saw mothers on drugs as a danger to their babies, and we kept them away from here. Just recently I became angry with a woman for taking drugs during her pregnancy. She was turning her baby into an addict. Her own baby! I wanted to slap her, but I controlled my anger. I told her that she should hold the baby because it was experiencing stress. Maybe it was the touch of that helpless child; whatever, the mother entered a drug rehabilitation program. And she's doing okay."

Listening to Cindy, I recall an essay by the physician and philosopher Lewis Thomas. Its point is that the dismay of being sick comes in part from the loss of close human contact; touch is medicine's real professional secret.

Far from Parkland, at Beth Israel Hospital in Boston, I hear similar opinions from Dr. Thomas Delbanco, an internist who has taken a sabbatical from his practice to head the Picker/Commonwealth Program for Patient-Centered Care. The issue of illness as a life crisis for patient and family, Delbanco says, has been given too little attention in the medical community. New studies are suggesting that patients who receive information and emotional support fare better on the average than those who do not. According to these studies, closer contact between physicians and patients can improve the chances of a good recovery.

Delbanco comes from a family of artists and plays the violin, an instrument whose uniqueness he compares to each individual's experience of illness. "There are two important parts of me," he says. "There is the physician and there is the musician. Music connects me with the importance of being replenished spiritually. And that is something that as a physician I must never forget. The patient before me is a human being with the same joys, sorrows, and complexities as myself. Doctors have to listen to what makes one person different from the other and constantly evaluate that distinction in order to figure out what makes one treatment work better for one person and not the other."

He introduces our team to Audrey and Ed Taylor. Audrey, who is fifty-eight, works in computer graphics. She is about to experience one of the most traumatic events in medicine—open heart surgery. Dr. Delbanco will follow her through the experience and interpret it for her and her family: her husband, Ed, a retired firefighter; their son, Ed, Jr., an MIT graduate with a degree in engineering, who now runs his own small construction company; and their daughter, Ruthie, an elementary-school teacher. Audrey's ordeal will test the family. How they manage their collective trauma, Delbanco explains, can affect Audrey's recovery from the surgery. "The hospitalization of a loved one is a crisis for the whole family. Families can interfere with medicine or they can be the medicine. I would say that respecting and facilitating family bonds may be more crucial to a patient's survival than the latest diagnostic procedure or therapeutic innovation. All too often they are left out of the picture. As doctors, we don't get into the house anymore. And we don't get that larger context in the examining room.

"If we physicians also thought of ourselves as medicine," he says, "we would treat people differently. The more informed you are as a patient and the more your family understands what is happening, the more you and they will be able to make wiser decisions. Information is hope. The terrible doctor robs the patient of hope. As physicians, we have to treat the body and appeal to the mind—the patient's and the family's."

This rings true to me. When I was growing up, our family doctor in Marshall, Texas, instinctively knew a lot about healing and the mind. When he asked, "How are you feeling?" he was interested in more than our stomachaches or fevers. He lived down the street, went to the church on the corner, knew where my parents worked, knew our relatives and family history—and he knew how to listen. He treated the patient holistically before anyone there ever heard of the term.

That was years ago. Today the practice of medicine in an urban,

Love cures people—both the ones who give it and the ones who receive it.

—Karl A. Menninger

technological society rarely provides either the time or the environment to encourage a doctor-patient relationship that promotes healing. Many modern doctors also lack the requisite training for this kind of healing. As Eric J. Cassell writes in *The Nature Of Suffering and the Goals of Medicine*, "Without system and training, being responsive in the face of suffering remains the attribute of individual physicians who have come to this mastery alone or gained it from a few inspirational teachers." Healing powers, Cassell continues, "consist only in and no more than in allowing, causing, or bringing to bear those things or forces for getting better (whatever they may be) that already exist in the patient." The therapeutic instrument in this healing is "indisputably" the doctor, whose power flows not from control over the patient but from his or her own self-mastery. Modern physicians have mastered admirably the power of the latest scientific medicine. To excel at the art of healing requires the same systematic discipline.

Talking with different doctors during this journey, I realize that we do need a new medical paradigm that goes beyond "body parts" medicine, and not only for the patient's sake. At a time when the cost of health care is skyrocketing, the potential economic impact of mind/body medicine is considerable. Thinking about our medical system as a "health care" system rather than a "disease treatment" system would mean looking closely at medical education and our public funding priorities.

On this first stage of my journey, I realize that the subject of healing and the mind stretches beyond medicine into issues about what we value in society and who we are as human beings. As patients, we are more than lonely, isolated flecks of matter; we are members of families, communities, and cultures. As this awareness finds its way into hospitals, operating rooms, clinics, and doctors' offices, perhaps it will spread further, as well. Healing begins with caring. So does civilization.

Much of our capacity to help another person depends upon our state of mind. Sometimes our minds are so scattered, confused, depressed, or agitated, we can hardly get out of bed. At other times we're clear, alert, and receptive; we feel ready, even eager, to respond generously to the needs of others.

—Ram Dass and Paul Gorman

T H E   U S E   O F   F O R C E

William Carlos Williams

T HEY WERE NEW PATIENTS TO ME, ALL I HAD WAS THE NAME, OLSON. PLEASE COME DOWN AS SOON AS YOU CAN, my daughter is very sick.

When I arrived I was met by the mother, a big startled looking woman, very clean and apologetic who merely said, Is this the doctor? and let me in. In the back, she added. You must excuse us, doctor, we have her in the kitchen where it is warm. It is very damp here sometimes.

The child was fully dressed and sitting on her father's lap near the kitchen table. He tried to get up, but I motioned for him not to bother, took off my overcoat and started to look things over. I could see that they were all very nervous, eyeing me up and down distrustfully. As often, in such cases, they weren't telling me more than they had to, it was up to me to tell them; that's why they were spending three dollars on me.

The child was fairly eating me up with her cold, steady eyes, and no expression to her face whatever. She did not move and seemed, inwardly, quiet; an unusually attractive little thing, and as strong as a heifer in appearance. But her face was flushed, she was breathing rapidly, and I realized that she had a high fever. She had magnificent blonde hair, in profusion. One of those picture children often reproduced in advertising leaflets and the photogravure sections of the Sunday papers.

She's had a fever for three days, began the father and we don't know what it comes from. My wife has

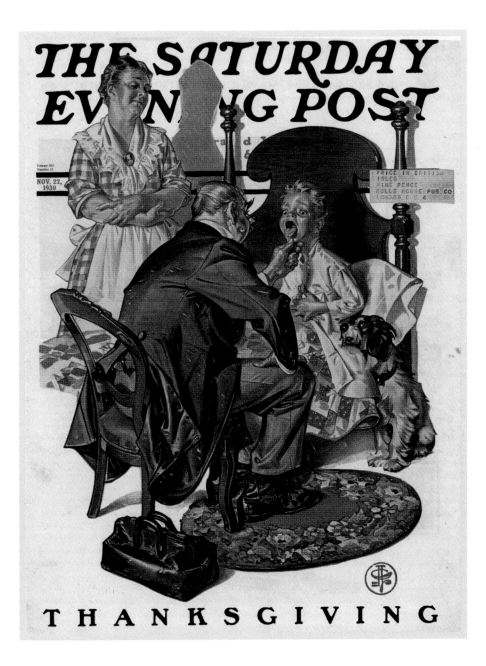

given her things, you know, like people do, but it don't do no good. And there's been a lot of sickness around. So we tho't you'd better look her over and tell us what is the matter.

As doctors often do I took a trial shot at it as a point of departure. Has she had a sore throat?

Both parents answered me together, No . . . No, she says her throat don't hurt her.

Does your throat hurt you? added the mother to the child. But the little girl's expression didn't change nor did she move her eyes from my face.

Have you looked?

I tried to, said the mother, but I couldn't see.

As it happens we had been having a number of cases of diphtheria in the school to which this child went during that month and we were all, quite apparently, thinking of that, though no one had as yet spoken of the thing.

Well, I said, suppose we take a look at the throat first. I smiled in my best professional manner and asking for the child's first name I said, come on, Mathilda, open your mouth and let's take a look at your throat.

Nothing doing.

Aw, come on, I coaxed, just open your mouth wide and let me take a look. Look, I said opening both hands wide, I haven't anything in my hands. Just open up and let me see.

Such a nice man put in the mother. Look how kind he is to you. Come on, do what he tells you to. He won't hurt you.'

At that I ground my teeth in disgust. If only they wouldn't use the word "hurt" I might be able to get somewhere. But I did not allow myself to be hurried or disturbed but speaking quietly and slowly I approached the child again.

As I moved my chair a little nearer suddenly with one cat-like movement both her hands clawed instinctively for my eyes and she almost reached them too. In fact she knocked my glasses flying and they fell, though unbroken, several feet away from me on the kitchen floor.

Both the mother and father almost turned themselves inside out in embarrassment and apology. You bad girl, said the mother, taking her and shaking her by one arm. Look what you've done. The nice man. . . .

For heaven's sake, I broke in. Don't call me a nice man to her. I'm here to look at her throat on the chance that she might have diphtheria and possibly die of it. But that's nothing to her. Look here, I said to the child, we're going to look at your throat. You're old enough to understand what I'm saying. Will you open it now by yourself or shall we have to open it for you?

Not a move. Even her expression hadn't changed. Her breaths however were coming faster and faster. Then the battle began. I had to do it. I had to have a throat culture for her own protection. But first I told the parents that it was entirely up to them. I explained the danger but said that I would not insist on a throat examination so long as they would take the responsibility.

If you dent do what the doctor says you'll have to go to the hospital, the mother admonished her severely.

Oh yeah? I had to smile to myself. After all, I had already fallen in love with the savage brat, the parents were contemptible to me. In the ensuing struggle they grew more and more abject, crushed, exhausted, while she surely rose to magnificent heights of insane fury of effort bred of her terror of me.

The father tried his best, and he was a big man but the fact that she was his daughter, his shame at her behavior and his dread of hurting her made him release her just at the critical moment several times when I had almost achieved success, till I wanted to kill him. But his dread also that she might have diphtheria made him tell me to go on, go on though he himself was almost fainting, while the mother moved back and forth behind us raising and lowering her hands in an agony of apprehension.

Put her in front of you on your lap, I ordered, and hold both her wrists.

But as soon as he did the child let out a scream. Don't, you're hurting me. Let go of my hands. Let them go I tell you. Then she shrieked terrifyingly hysterically. Stop it! stop it! You're killing me!

Do you think she can stand it, doctor! said the mother.

You get out, said the husband to his wife. Do you want her to die of diphtheria?

Come on now, hold her, I said.

Then I grasped the child's head with my left hand and tried to get the wooden tongue depressor between her teeth. She fought, with clenched teeth, desperately! But now I also had grown furious—at a child. I tried to hold myself down but I couldn't. I know how to expose a throat for inspection. And I did my best. When finally I got the wooden spatula behind the last teeth and just the point of it into the mouth cavity, she opened up for an instant but before I could see anything she came down again and gripping the wooden blade between her molars she reduced it to splinters before I could get it out again.

Aren't you ashamed, the mother yelled at her. Aren't you ashamed to act like that in front of the doctor?

Get me a smooth-handled spoon of some sort, I told the mother. We're going through with this.

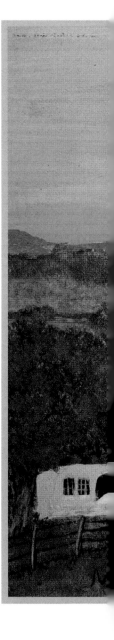

The child's mouth was already bleeding. Her tongue was cut and she was screaming in wild hysterical shrieks. Perhaps I should have desisted and come back in an hour or more. No doubt it would have been better. But I have seen at least two children lying dead in bed of neglect in such cases, and feeling that I must get a diagnosis now or never I went at it again. But the worst of it was that I too had got beyond reason, I could have torn the child apart in my own fury and enjoyed it. It was a pleasure to attack her. My face was burning with it.

The damned little brat must be protected against her own idiocy, one says to one says to one's self at such times. Others must be protected against her. It is social necessity. And all these things are true. But a blind fury, a feeling of adult shame, bred of a longing for muscular release are the operatives. One goes on to the end.

In a final unreasoning assault I overpowered the child's neck and jaws. I forced the heavy silver spoon back of her teeth and down her throat till she gagged. And there it was— both tonsils covered with membrane. She had fought valiantly to keep me from knowing her secret. She had been hiding that sore throat for three days at least and lying to her parents in order to escape just such an outcome as this.

Now truly she *was* furious. She had been on the defensive before but now she attacked. Tried to get off her father's lap and fly at me while tears of defeat blinded her eyes.

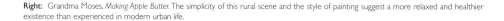

Right: Grandma Moses, *Making Apple Butter.* The simplicity of this rural scene and the style of painting suggest a more relaxed and healthier existence than experienced in modern urban life.

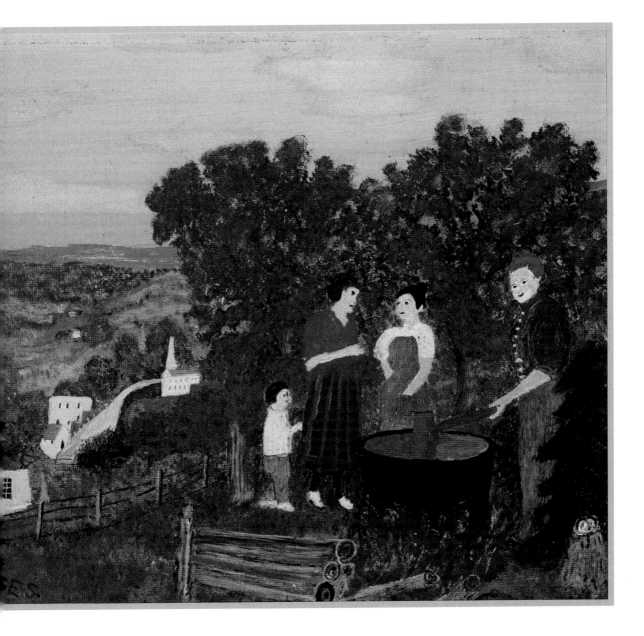

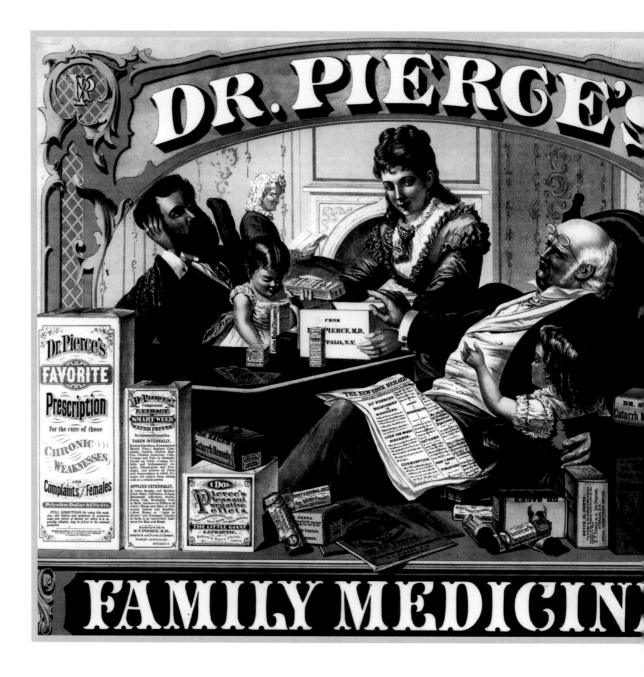

HOUSE CALLS

Lewis Thomas

M<small>Y FATHER TOOK ME ALONG ON HOUSE CALLS WHENEVER</small> I <small>WAS AROUND THE HOUSE, ALL</small> through my childhood. He liked company, and I liked watching him and listening to him. This must have started when I was five years old, for I remember riding in the front seat from one house to another, and back and forth from the hospital, when my father and many of the people on the streets were wearing gauze masks; it was the 1918 influenza epidemic.

One of the frequent calls which I found fascinating was at a big house on Sanford Avenue; he never parked the car in front of this house, but usually left it, and me, a block away around the corner. Later, he explained that the patient was a prominent Christian Scientist, a pillar of that church. He could perfectly well have parked in front if there had been a clearer understanding all around of what he was up to, for it was, in its way, faith healing.

I took the greatest interest in his doctor's bag, a miniature black suitcase, fitted inside to hold his stethoscope and various glass bottles and ampules, syringes and needles, and a small metal case for instruments. It smelled of Lysol and ether. All he had in the bag was a handful of things. Morphine was the most important, and the only really

Left: A medicine advertisement from 1874 when treatment was much more home-based.

indispensable drug in the whole pharmacopoeia. Digitalis was next in value. Insulin had arrived by the time he had been practicing for twenty years, and he had it. Adrenalin was there, in small glass ampules, in case he ran into a case of anaphylactic shock; he never did. As he drove his rounds, he talked about the patients he was seeing.

I'm quite sure my father always hoped I would want to become a doctor, and that must have been part of the reason for taking me along on his visits. But the general drift of his conversation was intended to make clear to me, early on, the aspect of medicine that troubled him most all through his professional life; there were so many people needing help, and so little that he could do for any of them. It was necessary for him to be available, and to make all these calls at their homes, but I was not to have the idea that he could do anything much to change the course of their illnesses. It was important to my father that I understand this; it was a central feature of the profession, and a doctor should not only be prepared for it but be even more prepared to be honest with himself about it.

It was not always easy to be honest, he said. One of his first patients, who had come to see him in his new office when he was an unknown in town, was a man complaining of grossly bloody urine. My father examined him at length, took a sample of the flawed urine, did a few other tests, and found himself without a diagnosis. To buy time enough to read up on the matter, he gave the patient a bottle of Blaud's pills, a popular iron remedy for anemia at the time, and told him to come back to the office in four days. The patient returned on the appointed day jubilant, carrying a flask of crystal-clear urine, totally cured. In the following months my father discovered that his reputation had been made by this therapeutic triumph. The word was out, all over town, that that new doctor, Thomas, had gifts beyond his own knowledge—this last because my father's outraged protests that his Blaud's pills could have had nothing whatever to do with recovery from bloody urine. The man had probably passed a silent kidney stone and that was all there was to it, said my father. But he had already gained the reputation of a healer, and it grew through all the years of his practice, and there was nothing he could do about it.

Even now, twenty-five years after his death, I meet people from time to time who lived once in Flushing, or whose parents lived there, and I hear the same anecdotes about his abilities: children with meningitis or rheumatic fever whose lives had been saved by him, patients with pneumonia who had recovered under his care, even people with incurable endocarditis, overwhelming typhoid fever, peritonitis, what-all.

But the same stories are told about any good, hardworking general practitioner of that day. Patients do get better, some of them anyway, from even the worst diseases; there are very few illnesses, like rabies, that kill all comers. Most of them tend to kill some patients and spare others, and if you are one of the lucky ones and have also had at hand a steady, knowledgeable doctor, you become convinced that the doctor saved you. My father's early instructions to me, sitting in the front of his car on his rounds, were that I should be careful not to believe this of myself if I became a doctor.

Nevertheless, despite his skepticism, he carried his prescription pad everywhere and wrote voluminous prescriptions for all his patients. These were fantastic formulations, containing five or six different vegetable ingredients, each one requiring careful measuring and weighing by the druggist, who pounded the powder, dissolved it in alcohol, and bottled it with a label giving only the patient's name, the date, and the instructions about dosage. The contents were a deep mystery, and intended to be a mystery. The prescriptions were always written in Latin, to heighten the mystery. The purpose of this kind of therapy was essentially reassurance. A skilled, experienced physician might have dozens of different formulations in his memory, ready for writing out in flawless detail at a moment's notice, but all he could have predicted about them with any certainty were the variations in the degree of bitterness of taste, the color, the smell, and the likely effects of the concentrations of alcohol used as solvent. They were placebos, and they had been the principal mainstay of medicine, the sole technology, for so long a time—millennia—that they had the incantatory power of religious ritual. My father had little faith in the effectiveness of any of them, but he used them daily in his practice. They were expected by his patients; a doctor who did not provide such prescriptions would soon have no practice at all; they did no harm, so far as he could see; if nothing else, they gave the patient something to do while the illness, whatever, was working its way through its appointed course.

The United States Pharmacopoeia, an enormous book, big as the family Bible, stood on a bookshelf in my father's office, along with scores of textbooks and monographs on medicine and surgery. The ingredients that went into the prescriptions, and the recipes for their compounding and administration, were contained in the *Pharmacopoeia*. There was no mistaking the earnestness of that volume; it was a thousand pages of true belief: this set of ingredients was useful in pulmonary tuberculosis, that one in "acute indigestion" (the term then used for what later turned out to be coronary thrombosis), another in neurasthenia (weak nerves; almost all patients had weak nerves, one time or another), and so on, down through the known catalogue of human ailments. There was a different prescription for every circumstance, often three or four. The most popular and widely used ones were the "tonics," good for bucking up the spirits; these contained the headiest concentrations

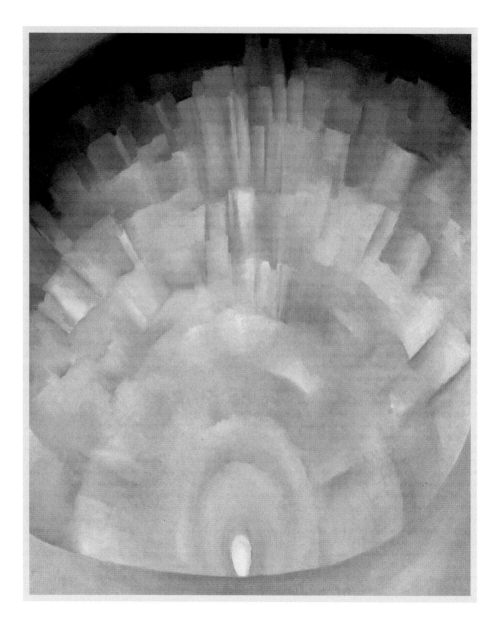

of alcohol. Opium had been the prime ingredient in the prescriptions of the nineteenth century, edited out when it was realized that great numbers of elderly people, especially, "nervous" women, were sitting in their rocking chairs, addicted beyond recall.

The tradition still held when I was a medical student at Harvard. In the outpatient department of the Boston City Hospital, through which hundreds of patients filed each day for renewal of their medications, each doctor's desk had a drawerful of prescriptions already printed out to save time, needing only the doctor's signature. The most popular one, used for patients with chronic, obscure complaints, was *Elixir of I, Q ,and S*, iron, quinine, and strychnine, each ingredient present in tiny amounts, dissolved in the equivalent of bourbon.

Medicine was subject to recurrent fads in therapy throughout my father's career. Long before his time, homeopathy emerged and still had many devout practitioners during his early years; this complex theory, involving what was believed to be the therapeutic value of "like versus like," and the administration of minuscule quantities of drugs that imitated the symptoms of the illness in question, took hold in the mid-nineteenth century in reaction against the powerfully toxic drugs then in common use—mercury, arsenic, bismuth, strychnine, aconite, and the like. Patients given the homeopathic drugs felt better and had a better chance of surviving, about the same as they would have had without treatment, and the theory swept the field for many decades.

A new theory, attributing all human disease to the absorption of toxins from the lower intestinal tract, achieved high fashion in the first decade of this century. "Autointoxication" became the fundamental disorder to be overcome by treatment, and the strongest measures were introduced to empty the large bowel and keep it empty. Cathartics, ingenious variations of the enema, and other devices for stimulating peristalsis took over medical therapy. My father, under persuasion by a detail man from one of the medical supply houses, purchased one of these in 1912, a round lead object the size of a bowling ball, encased in leather. This was to be loaned to the patient, who was instructed to lie flat in bed several times daily and roll it clockwise around the abdomen, following the course of the colon. My father tried it for a short while on a few patients, with discouraging results, and one day placed it atop a cigar box which he had equipped with wheels and a long string, and presented it to my eldest sister, who tugged it with pleasure around the corner to a neighbor's house. That was the last he saw of the ball until twelve years later, when the local newspaper announced in banner headlines that a

Left: Georgia O'Keeffe, *Abstraction—White Rose III.*

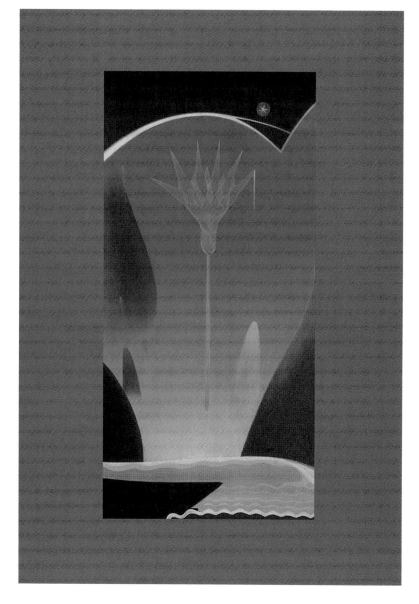

Left: Agnes Pelton, *Lotus for Lida.* The artist considered this an image of renewal and rejuvenation, and it recalls how the woman in the text finds rejuvenation, albeit in an unusual way.

CUPID'S DISEASE

Oliver Sacks

A BRIGHT WOMAN OF NINETY, NATASHA K., RECENTLY CAME TO OUR CLINIC. SOON AFTER HER EIGHTY-EIGHTH birthday, she said, she noticed 'a change.' What sort of change? we queried.

'Delightful!' she exclaimed. 'I thoroughly enjoyed it. I felt more energetic, more alive—I felt young once again. I took all interest in the young men. I started to feel, you might say, "frisky"—yes, frisky.'

'This was a problem?'

'No, not at first. I felt well, *extremely* well—why should I think anything was the matter?'

'And then?'

'My friends started to worry. First they said, "You look radiant—a new lease on life!", but then they started to think it was not quite—appropriate. "You were always so shy," they said, "and now you're a flirt. You giggle, you tell jokes—at your age, is that right?"

'And how did you feel?'

'I was taken aback. I'd been carried along, and it didn't occur to me to question what was happening. But then I did. I said to myself, "You're 89, Natasha, this has been going on for a year. You were always so temperate in feeling—and now this extravagance! You are all old woman, nearing the end. What could justify such a sudden euphoria?" And as soon as I thought of euphoria, things took on a new complexion . . . "You're sick, my dear," I said to myself. "You're feeling *too* well, you have to be ill!"

'Ill? Emotionally? Mentally ill?'

'No, not emotionally—physically ill. It was something in my body, my brain, that was making me high. And then I thought—goddam it, it's Cupid's Disease!'

'Cupid's Disease?' I echoed, blankly. I had never heard of the term before.

'Yes, Cupid's Disease—syphilis, you know. I was in a brothel in Salonika, nearly seventy years ago. I caught syphilis—lots of the girls had it—we called it Cupid's Disease. My husband saved me, took me out, had it treated. That was years before penicillin, of course. Could it have caught up with me after all these years?'

There may be an immense latent period between the primary infection and the advent of neurosyphilis, especially if the primary infection has been suppressed, not eradicated. I had one patient, treated with Salvarsan by Ehrlich himself, who developed *tabes dorsalis*—one form of neurosyphilis—more than fifty years later.

But I had never heard of an interval of *seventy years*—nor of a self-diagnosis of cerebral syphilis mooted so calmly and clearly.

'That's an amazing suggestion,' I replied after some thought. 'It would never have occurred to me, but perhaps you are right.'

She was right; the spinal fluid was positive, she did have neurosyphilis, it *was* indeed the spirochetes stimulating her ancient cerebral cortex. Now the question of treatment arose. But here another dilemma presented itself, propounded, with typical acuity, by Mrs. K. herself. 'I don't know that I *want* it treated,' she said. 'I know it's an illness, but it's made me feel *well*. I've enjoyed it, I still enjoy it, I won't deny it. It's made me feel livelier, friskier, than I have in twenty years. It's been fun. But I know when a good thing goes too far, and stops being good. I've had thoughts, I've had impulses, I won't tell you, which are—well, embarrassing and silly. It was like being a little tiddly, a little tipsy, at first, but if it goes any further . . .' She mimed a drooling, spastic dement. 'I guessed I had Cupid's, that's why I came to you. I don't want it to get worse, that would be awful; but I don't want it cured—that would be just as bad. I wasn't fully alive until the wrigglies got me. *Do you think you could keep it just as it is?*'

We thought for a while, and our course, mercifully, was clear. We have given her penicillin, which has killed the spirochetes, but can do nothing to reverse the cerebral changes, the disinhibitions, they have caused.

And now Mrs. K. has it both ways, enjoying a mild disinhibition, a release of thought and impulse, without any threat to her self-control or of further damage to her cortex. She hopes to live, thus reanimated, rejuvenated, to a hundred. 'Funny thing,' she says. 'You've got to give it to Cupid.'

Right: Charles Burchfield, *Woodpecker*. Burchfield's painting shows his incredible ability to convey nature's vibrancy, which mirrors the aliveness of the woman in the story.

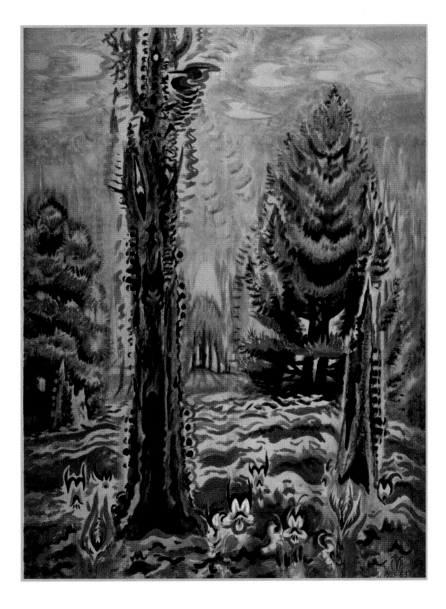

D O C T O R , T A L K T O M E

Anatole Broyard

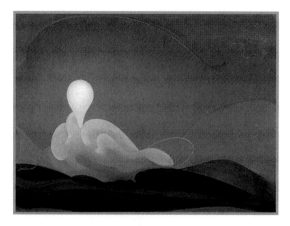

HEN, IN THE SUMMER OF 1989, I MOVED from Connecticut to Cambridge, Massachusetts, I found that I had difficulty urinating. I was like Portnoy, in *Portnoy's Complaint*, who couldn't fornicate in Israel. I had always wanted to live in Cambridge, and the thought passed through my mind that I couldn't urinate because—like Israel for Portnoy—Cambridge was a transcendent place for me.

When my inhibition persisted, I began to think about a doctor, and I set about finding one in the superstitious manner most of us fall back on: I asked a couple I knew for a recommendation. To be recommended, for whatever unreasonable reasons, gives a doctor an aura, a history, a shred of magic. Though I thought of my disorder as a simple matter—prostatitis is common in men of my age—I still wanted a potent doctor.

I applied to this particular couple for a recommendation because they are the two most critical people I know: critics of philosophy, politics, history, literature, drama, music. They are the sort of people for whom information is a religion, and the rigor of their conversation is legendary. To talk with them is an ordeal, a fatigue of fine distinctions, and I wanted a doctor who had survived such a scrutiny.

Above: Agnes Pelton, *Sea Change.*   **Right:** Carl Gustav Jung (1875-1961). Jung was the first to formulate the idea of archetypes and, of course, was also a prime advocate of the benefits of listening to patients.

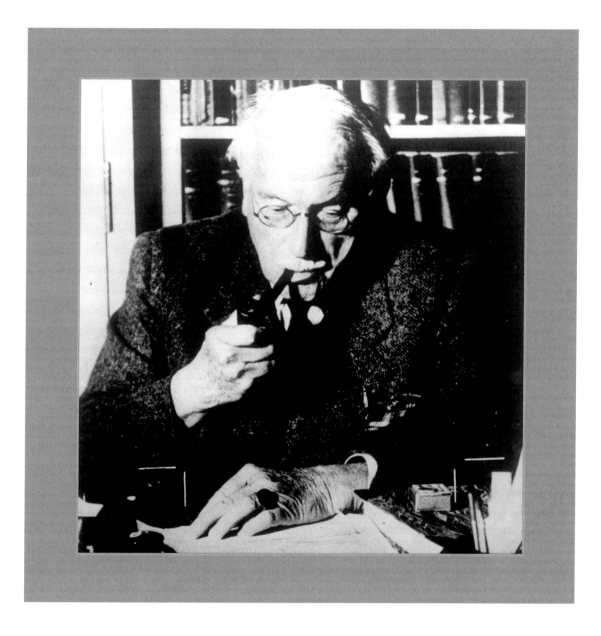

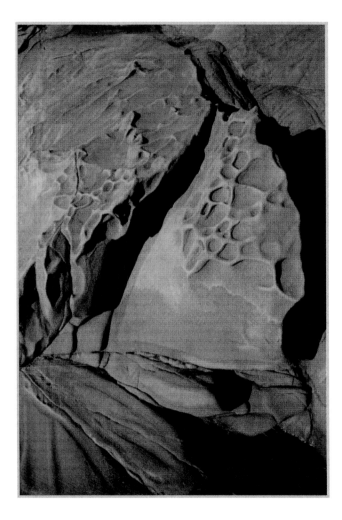

T O U C H I N G

David Hellerstein

S COOT DOWN TO THE EDGE OF THE
table, hon," says Dr. Snarr. The
small room is hot, the air stuffy.
Our patient winces at the word *hon*. She
is a young woman with chronic pelvic
pain, the bane of gynecologists, and I can
tell she doesn't like Snarr's tone. She does
scoot along the table, though, and Snarr
kicks a wheeled stool toward me. I sit on
it, slide between her legs, ready for my

Left: Photograph of rocks at Bean Hollow on the California
coast. The rock formations in this photograph show their
responsiveness to the environment, no matter how hard they
are they have been shaped by wind and erosion—unhappily
the doctor in the story does not.

lesson of the day. Feet and calves and thighs surround me, suddenly very close. Snarr positions the lamp before my chest, so light pours on her. I warm the speculum in my gloved hand and, with a twist, insert it.

"Open it up," he says. "Tighten it all the way open. Pull down to keep away from the urethra, You hit the urethra and no patient will ever come back to you."

Snarr is my teacher, a gaunt and narrow-shouldered man with a small potbelly below the belt of his corduroy pants. Before coming in here, he went over the information I had gathered and insisted it was nonsense. She couldn't possibly feel that kind of pain. I must not be asking the right questions. Hadn't I learned anything? Gynecologists traditionally have the reputation of being the dummies of medicine: surgeons laugh at their clumsiness in the operating room, internists at their ignorance of medical fact, psychiatrists at their insensitivity. And so far Snarr had done nothing to dispel that prejudice, which was too bad, considering that I was an impressionable third-year medical student, still trying to decide what field to select.

"Okay," says Snarr. "Now swab it out real well. Get some cells on that."

I swab.

"Pull that speculum out now. Get a good look at those walls."

I see pink folds as I pull, pink, moist walls bulging against the metal of the speculum—aquatic territory, the scalloped forms of submarine life. It's out. Snarr is quick next with lubricating jelly on the first two fingers of my glove. I stand up, push the stool away. I begin the manual exam.

"*Aiee!*" The woman screams and slides up on the table. "God! Oh God!"

"So that's. . . that's where it hurts," I say. I'm sweating. "Just. . . just a second, I'll try more gently."

I feel around again. This time she doesn't scream. She breathes deeply. I can't feel a damn thing, but with Snarr watching I can't pull out right away. For a month I've been spending afternoons in the gynecology clinic with Dr. Snarr—a month of women's bottoms on the edges of tables, of the hot lamp in front of my chest, the examining glove on my hand, powdered inside, the smells of femaleness. And the confidences of women, fascinating and at times overpowering, about their pains, their periods, their fertility, their husbands, their lovers. What gets to me, though, are the exams. The touching. Deep internal touching, feeling for the bulge of the uterus, for those small elusive olives the ovaries, exploring for tenderness, creating sudden moments of pain. Technically I'm reasonably good, as good as can be expected for a third-year medical student rotating through Ob-Gyn. But I still find it strange to be touching intimately but without passion—as a doctor.

I'm not alone in this either; the other medical students on Ob-Gyn seem just as awkward as I. We hang around in the lounge, where the pharmaceutical rep sometimes leaves free coffee and doughnuts, cracking jokes, laughing too much.

It reminds me of another situation, in the second-year physical diagnosis course, where we had to examine each other. The new idea that year was that we'd learn how to be more compassionate doctors if we practiced physical exams on one another first, before going on to patients.

We were divided into small groups, men and women together, and sent to various examining rooms. Our exams began at the head and worked down. You couldn't get too upset about looking into your medical student buddy's eyes, but by the second session, when we got down to the chest, the protests began. First the women complained and refused to be examined, but as it became clear that genital and rectal exams were also part of the required curriculum, men started to protest as well. Finally there was a full-scale revolt. A petition was circulated, meetings were hurriedly arranged with various administrators, protests were loud and vocal. The class was boycotted. We ended up learning the pelvic exam on professional models and doing rectal exams on plastic dummies. No one felt the course should be repeated.

I've always been sort of puzzled why my fellow medical students got so upset. After all, we had done just about everything together—cut open cadavers, crammed for exams, played touch football on the front lawn, dated and flirted and confided and complained. What it comes down to, I think, was that after two years together in med school, we knew each other too well, far too well for touching to be neutral. To palpate, percuss, auscultate, and probe each other's bodies brought out too many undoctorly thoughts.

We were a long way, I realize now, from learning the doctor's dispassionate touch. But the real problem came when our teachers were no better than we—when they were clumsy and awkward, too.

"All right," Dr. Snarr says, "let me try my hand." He steps in. I strip off my glove and wash my hands, ready to observe a deft exam, pinpointing the source of pain, exploring yet reassuring.

But in a second the woman is screaming, writhing on the table. Snarr is reaching way far in, clumsily it seems, pushing so hard her hips rise from the table; and she is crying, grabbing the table with her hands. I feel sick just watching. I have no way of knowing what, if anything, Snarr is finding, since he does not explain.

"All right, hon," he tells her. He pulls off his glove. "Wipe yourself off; we'll come back and see you in a minute."

"I don't know why the heck she hurts," he says when we are outside. "Give her some estrogen cream."

She'd dressed when I come back in. She's pale and woozy, and there's still pain in her eyes. I hand her the prescription.

"Come back if it gets worse," I say.

"Than what?" the woman asks.

I am embarrassed. I murmur something, that I'm sorry we didn't come up with anything. Then I hurry out after my teacher,

I find him in the side room, having coffee and doughnuts, courtesy of the pharmaceutical rep. The next patient isn't ready yet.

"Have some," he says.

I decline. I'm too jittery to eat.

"That girl," says Dr. Snarr. "What do you think her problem is?"

I consider the possibilities: pelvic inflammatory disease, endometriosis, cysts. I talk, but I don't say what I really think: that he has no sense of what he put her through. That he's insensitive. Clumsy. A jerk. I'm disappointed, too, but I'm not sure why.

Perhaps it's that I wished he was a better doctor, a better role model. Certainly not all gynecologists are like Dr. Snarr, but at that moment it seemed as though they were. And what I needed so much was to know how to be with patients, how to deal with the feelings they evoked, how to make them feel at ease. If Dr. Snarr had been a better teacher, I might conceivably have gone into his field.

Dr. Snarr washes down the rest of his doughnut.

"So what else have we got out there?" he says.

A young black woman in a white gown looks around nervously as we enter.

"Scoot down to the edge of the table, hon," says Snarr.

Wincing at the word hon, the woman nevertheless scoots down.

Snarr kicks the wheeled stool over toward me.

And I begin.

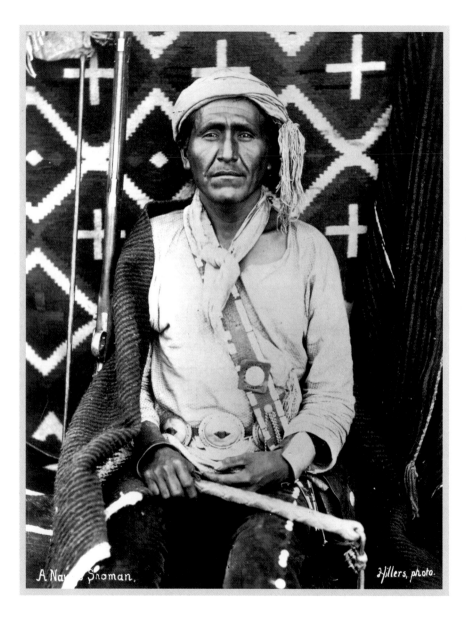

A Navajo Shaman.   Hillers, photo.

THE HEALING WATERS

Native American Myth

T HE IROQUOIS HAVE A TOUCHING STORY OF HOW A BRAVE OF THEIR RACE ONCE SAVED HIS WIFE AND HIS PEOPLE from extinction.

It was winter, the snow lay thickly on the ground, and there was sorrow in the encampment, for with the cold weather a dreadful plague had visited the people. There was not one but had lost some relative, and in some cases whole families had been swept away. Among those who had been most sorely bereaved was Nekumonta, a handsome young brave, who parents, brothers, sisters and children had died one by one before his eyes, while he was powerless to help them. And now his wife, the beautiful Shanewis, was weak and ill. The dreaded disease had laid its awful finger on her brow, and she knew that she must shortly bid her husband farewell and take her departure for the place of the dead. Already she saw her dead friends beckoning to her and inviting her to join them, but it grieved her terribly to think that she must leave her young husband in sorrow and loneliness. His despair was piteous to behold when she broke the sad news to him, but after the first outburst of grief he bore up bravely, and determined to fight the plague with all his strength.

Left: John K. Hillers, *Navaho Shaman.*

"I must find the healing herbs which the Great Manitou has planted," said he. "Wherever they may be, I must find them."

So he made his wife comfortable on her couch, covering her with warm furs, and the, embracing her gently, he set out on his difficult mission.

All day he sought eagerly in the forest for the healing herbs, but everywhere the snow lay deep, and not so much as a blade of grass was visible. When night came he crept along the frozen ground, thinking that his sense of smell might aid him in his search. Thus for three days and nights he wandered through the forest, over hills and across rivers, in a vain attempt to discover the means of curing the malady of Shanewis.

When he met a little scurrying rabbit in the path he cried eagerly: "Tell me, where shall I find the herbs which Manitou has planted?"

But the rabbit hurried away without reply, for he knew that the herbs had not yet risen above the ground, and he was very sorry for the brave.

Nekumonta came by and by to the den of a big bear, and of this animal also he asked the same question. But the bear could give him no reply, and he was obliged to resume his weary journey. He consulted all the beasts of the forest in turn, but from none could he get any help. How could they tell him, indeed, that his search was hopeless?

On the third night he was very weak and ill, for he had tasted no food since he had first set out, and he was numbed with cold and despair. He stumbled over a withered branch hidden under the snow, and so tired was he that he lay where he fell, and immediately went to sleep. All the birds and the beasts, all the multitude of creatures that inhabit the forest, came to watch over his slumbers. They remembered his kindness to them in former days, how he had never slain an animal unless he really needed it for food or clothing, how he had loved and protected the trees and the flowers. Their hearts were touched by his courageous fight for Shanewis, and they pitied his misfortunes. All that they could do to aid him they did. They cried to the Great Manitou to save his wife from the plague which held her, and the Great Spirit heard the manifold whispering and responded to their prayers.

While Nekumonta lay asleep there came to him the messenger of Manitou, and he dreamed. In his dream, he saw his beautiful Shanewis, pale and thin but as lovely as ever, and as he looked she smiled at him, and sang a strange, sweet song, like the murmuring of a distant waterfall. Then the scene changed, and it really was a waterfall he heard. In musical language it called him by name, saying: "See us, O Nekumonta, and when you find us Shanewis shall live. We are the Healing Waters of the Great Manitou."

Nekumonta awoke with the words of the song still ringing in his ears. Starting to his feet, he looked in every direction; but there was no water to be seen, though the murmuring sound of a waterfall was distinctly audible. He fancied he could even distinguish words in it.

"Release us!" it seemed to say. "Set us free, and Shanewis shall be saved!"

Nekumonta searched in vain for the waters. Then it suddenly occurred to him that they must be underground, directly under his feet. Seizing branches, stones, flints, he dug feverishly into the earth. So arduous was the task that before it was finished he was completely exhausted. But at last the hidden spring was disclosed and the waters were rippling merrily down the vale, carrying life and happiness wherever they went. The young man bathed his aching limbs in the healing stream, and in a moment he was well and strong.

Raising his hands, he gave thanks to Manitou. With eager fingers he made a jar of clay, and baked it in the fire, so that he might carry life to Shanewis. As he pursued his way homeward with his treasure his despair was changed to rejoicing and he sped like the wind.

When he reached his village his companions ran to greet him. Their faces were sad and hopeless, for the plague still raged. However, Nekumonta directed them to the Healing Waters and inspired them with new hope. Shanewis he found on the verge of the Shadow-land, and scarcely able to murmur a farewell to her husband. But Nekumonta did not listen to her broken adieux. He forced some of the Healing Water between her parched lips, and bathed her hands and her brow till she fell into a gentle slumber. When she awoke the fever had left her, she was serene and smiling, and Nekumonta's heart was filled with a great happiness.

The tribe was for ever rid of the dreaded plague, and the people gave to Nekumonta the title of 'Chief of the Healing Waters,' so that all might know that it was he who had brought them the gift of Manitou.

CANCER BECOMES ME

Marjorie Gross

S O I'M SITTING IN THE DOCTOR'S OFFICE, HE WALKS IN, JUST TELLS ME STRAIGHT OUT, "I WAS RIGHT—IT'S OVARIAN cancer, so I win. Pay up." And I say, "Oh, no, you're not gonna hold me to that, are you?" And he says, "Hey, a bet's a bet." You don't know what it's like to leave a doctor's office knowing you've lost a hundred dollars: suddenly everything's changed.

Well, OK, I've exaggerated a little. What really happens is the doctor walks in and gives you the sympathetic head tilt that right away tells you, "Don't buy in bulk." The degree of tilt corresponds directly with the level of bad news. You know, a little tilt: "We've caught it in time"; sixty-degree angle: "Spread to the lymph nodes"; forty-five-degree angle: "Spread to your clothes." In her book about cancer, Betty Rollin wrote, "First, you cry." However, she didn't mention what you do second, which is "Spend, spend, spend." You're sort of freed up, in a weird way. Suddenly, everything has a lifetime guarantee.

So I had a hysterectomy, and they found a tumor that they said was the size of an orange. (See, for women they use the citrus-fruit comparison; for men it's sporting goods: "Oh, it's the size of a softball." or, in England, a cricket ball.) I languished in the hospital for ten days, on a floor where everybody had cancer, so the sympathy playing field was level. You can't say, "Hey, can you keep it down? I just had my operation." You might get, "So what? I'm on my fifth." "Poor thing" doesn't really come into play much on this floor. My mother, who also had this disease (yeah, I inherited the cancer gene; my older brother got the blue eyes, but I'm not bitter)—

Right: Eliot Porter, *Apples on Tree After Frost*, Tesuques, New Mexico, November 21, 1966. Apples have long been symbolic of female sexuality, but in the photo they are frozen, a symbol recalling the woman in the story with ovarian cancer.

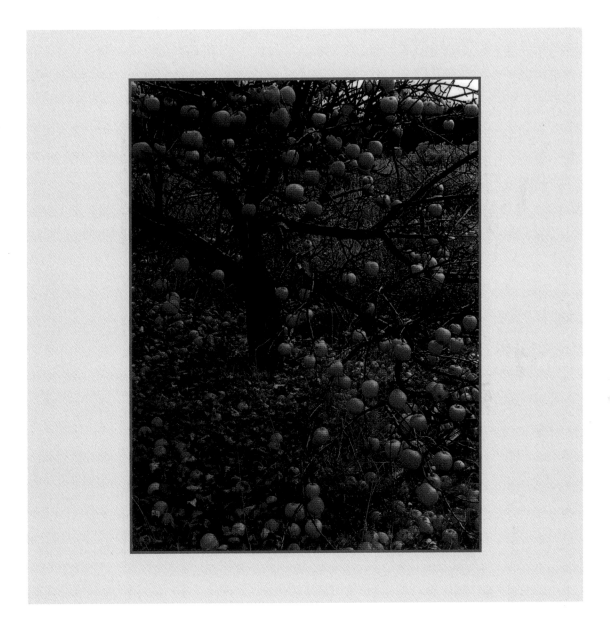

anyway, my mother told me that for some women a hospital stay is a welcome relief. You know, to have someone bringing you food, asking how you are, catering to your every vital sign. See, she wound up in a room with five other women, and they would sit around talking on one bed, and the minute the doctor walked in they would jump into their own beds and re-create the "incoming wounded" scene from "M*A*S*H," insuring that they would not be sent home early.

Which now leads us quixotically but inevitably to chemotherapy. What can I say about chemotherapy that hasn't already been said, in a million pop songs? I was prepared for the chemo side effects. I had my bald plans all in place. I decided to eschew wigs—all except the rainbow wig. Once in a while, I'd put that on when I didn't want to be stared at. Luckily, in my life-style (Lesbeterian) you can be bald and still remain sexually attractive. In fact, the word "sexy" has been thrown my way more times this year than ever before. I've had dreams where my hair grows back and I'm profoundly disappointed. The bald thing works on other levels as well. The shortened shower time—in and out in three minutes easy. Shampoo-free travel. Plus, I get to annoy my father for the first time in twenty years. He hates to see me flaunting my baldness. I thought I'd lost the power to disgust him, but it was right there under my follicles all along.

The other side effect is that I've lost twenty pounds, which has sent my women friends into spasms of jealousy. I think I even heard "Lucky stiff." I said, "I think I'm closer to being a stiff than lucky!" But it fell on deaf ears. I suppose it's a testament to the overall self-esteem of my fellow-women that, after hearing all about the operations, the chemo, and the nausea, the only thing that registers is "Wow, twenty pounds!" and "You look fabulous!" It's a really good weight-loss system for the terminally lazy. I mean, a StairMaster would have been preferable, but mine wound up as a pants tree.

Then, there are my other friends, who are bugging me to go alternative. So now I'm inundated with articles, books, and pamphlets on healers, nutritionists, and visualization (which I know doesn't work, because if it did, Uma Thurman would be running around my house naked asking me what I want for breakfast). I was also given a crystal by a friend who was going through a messy divorce. She was given the crystal by a guy who died of AIDS. As far as I was concerned, this crystal had a terrible résumé. As far as the healing power of crystals goes, let me just say that I grew up eating dinner under a crystal chandelier every night, and look what came of *that*: two cancers, a busted marriage and an autistic little brother. There, the healing power of crystals. Enjoy.

This is not to say I'm completely devoid of spirituality. I mean, when you're faced with the dark specter of death you formulate an afterlife theory in a hurry. I decided to go with reincarnation, mixed with some sort of Heaven-like holding area. Then, of course, we could also just turn to dust and that's it. I come from a family of dust believers. They believe in dust and money: the tangibles. The thing about death that bugs me the most is that I don't want to get there before all my friends. I don't even like to be the first one at the restaurant.

The hardest part of this whole thing is that it has completely ruined my loner lifestyle. I've never felt the need to have anyone around constantly. I mean, I never wear anything that zips up in the back, and I hate cowboy boots. And now I get ten times as many phone calls—people wanting to come over and see me. When I'm well, I can go months without seeing someone. Why the rush to see me nauseated? I especially don't believe in the hospital visit. People come in, you're lying there, you can't do anything, and they start talking about their plans for the night.

I hope with all this negative talk I haven't painted too bleak a picture and therefore discouraged you from getting cancer. I mean, there are some really good things about it. Like:

(1) You automatically get called courageous. The rest of you people have to save somebody from drowning. We just have to wake up.
(2) You are never called rude again. You can cancel appointments left and right, leave boring dinners after ten minutes, and still not become a social pariah.
(3) Everyone returns your calls immediately—having cancer is like being Mike Ovitz. And you're definitely not put on hold for long.
(4) People don't ask you to help them move.
(5) If you're really shameless, you never have to wait in line for anything again. Take off the hat and get whisked to the front.

So it hasn't been all bad. I've done things I never would have done before. I even got to go to Europe with a creamy-white pop star. I used to use the word "someday," but now I figure someday is for people with better gene pools.

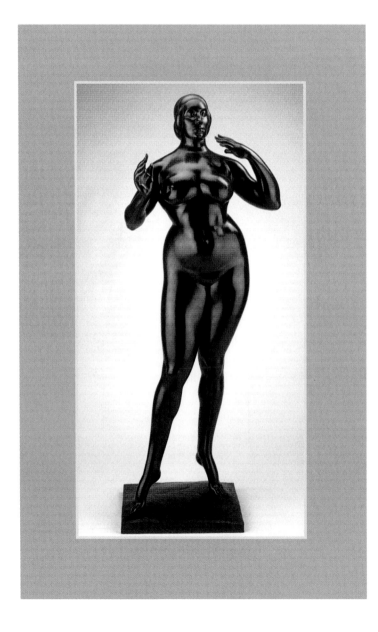

FAT

Carol Kloss

I SUCK HEAVY, SWEET, DARK SAUCE from chopped-up bones in the food court at the mall: baby back ribs from the Oriental Express, scraps of pork too charred to bite. While I eat, I watch people. A puffy-haired woman whose bottom and thighs droop off the seat of her chair. A saggy globe of a man with knees that will never touch and arms that can't hang straight; a skinny-legged little girl floats from

Left: Gaston Lachaise, *Standing Woman.*

the end of his hand. Three blocky women in shorts, no space between them and their big purses—boulders in the people-stream, their eyes focused on some solitary distance. We have each other, their faces say. I watch people and I watch fat: It rolls and jiggles under baggy shirts, shivers on over-bared thighs, swells the hand eating a sundae at the Dairy Queen.

"I hate cellulite," my husband told me once.

"Did you ever see your mother naked?" I asked.

"No, but there's such a thing as bathing suits," he said. "I dated a girl who was all cellulite; my mother fixed me up with her. She was just cellulite hanging on bones."

I watch the fat and wonder what's really inside, how deep it goes, how far away the bones are. Cushioned and pillowed, some people look boneless anyway, like boneless roasts, boneless pork roasts. Twist them slowly on a giant rotisserie and all the fat would drip off, dribble into the fire with every turn, drip and spurt and flame. Roast away all that fat—I'll take my gut well-done—and how much meat would be left? Maybe about as much as the shreds on the chopped-up Oriental Express bones. Maybe it depends on what you call the meat.

The fruit theory of fat says that pear fat is better than apple fat, this referring to the distribution of fat on the body: Store it in the legs and hips, not the belly, for less heart disease, cancer, diabetes, etc. Advertising and television and movies pick their bodies by the vegetable theory of fat: celery stalks. A lot of people are fruits trying to become vegetables, which is funny because most diets stuff you with vegetables and celery-stick nausea never dies. My mother-in-law, for instance, has been on a diet since 1962, and when she comes to my house for dinner she doesn't touch the salad.

Theory meets reality: Slap us in the diet pen, crack the whip of exercise, and pretty soon the calories counted and calories burned drift behind the television set while we cram into Slimmaire belts or ankle-length Spandex or blue jeans, the unisex girdle. Ah, support. That's what corsets were for. Where did they go? Maybe we should drag the whalebone out of the landfills. Or easier, order a floater from Lane Bryant, settle under your vertical-striped tent, and stay out of the wind.

Mostly we worry about it in guts, spare tires, balloon butts and saddlebags. But it also plumps cheeks, triples chins, inflates breasts, thickens ankles, and pads our feet and hands. Strip the skin from a pickled body and you'll see fat plastered everywhere, yellowed and chunky like margarine half-mixed with eggs. It bulges from the bottoms of kneecaps, hangs from arms and earlobes, swaddles the lymph nodes that cluster in armpits. The right coronary artery is wrapped in it, and the eyeballs lie on it.

Inside our nice coat of fat, with our little extra cushions tucked here and there, we have built-in protection from life's everyday shocks and jolts. Some people seem to need more protection than others. Like my friend Lana, a three-hundred-pound secretary who corrects her boss's grammar and improves his strategic plans but won't get a college degree. A person as fat as she, she says, couldn't go higher anyway. Or the man who lived in his bed except for the day he was supposed to leave on a free trip to Dick Gregory's fat farm. He got to the door but couldn't make himself go out and instead went back to the cushiony, crumb-covered pit of his specially reinforced mattress. Or my mother, who spent her days on a brown couch in a brown-carpeted room with brown-paneled walls, watching soap operas on a brown plastic television set. She built her protection from sardines and anchovies and pork and beans, cookies and day-old doughnuts and deep-fried onion rings. She dropped cigarette ash on her solitaire games and wrapped supper's potato peelings in the ads for the jobs she said she didn't know how to do.

Some fat is invisible. You see legs that look great in miniskirts; I see thighs that need the fat beaten out of them. You might think that you can get right up close and touch the edge of my size twelve body. But I feel the hidden tingle of my real edge a foot or two beyond your hand. The fat that you don't see tells me to strip my insides with laxatives and tells my husband's sister Trudi that she should only eat farina. It makes her wake her neighbors at four in the morning with the rumbling of her NordicTrack, and sometimes it throws her on the floor for 250 sit-ups while her parents watch from the dinner table. So, invisible fat has a lot of power. But it doesn't protect the back of Trudi's hand from her teeth when she shoves her finger down her throat. And it doesn't hide the sharpness of the shoulder blades that cut into my arms when I give her a hug.

Even though we try, we can't live without fat, and the more you have the luckier you are, really: all that adipose tissue bulging with future fatty acids, potential bits of muscle food, an internal portable Armageddon food cellar. If you happen to have accumulated an extra 220 pounds of it, you'd be able to live a theoretical year without going grocery shopping—quite a time-saver.

My grandmother swelled her fat cells with a special ethnic blend: Polish sausage fat, bacon fat, sour cream fat and cheesecake fat. About nine months of reserve lipids, I would guess she had, stored mostly between her neck and belly and carried around on fine muscled legs that her short, skinny beer-drinking husband admired. He died forty years before she did, and she fed five kids from the full-fat Polish meatcases in her three grocery stores. When she retired she became the baker for the St. John Berchmans bingo nights: cream cheese *kolacki* and deep-fried, jelly-filled *paczki* and all-butter poundcakes baked in pans so big that I was sure it would be a sin to keep a cake like that just for herself. She sold cheesecakes to her relatives and afghans to the priests. Then her doctor said she was too fat, and her daughters made her lose weight. When she got skinny she went into a nursing home, where she sat in a chair waiting for salt-free skinless chicken and begging quarters for the candy machine. And I brought her chocolate-frosted doughnuts from Amy Joy until she didn't remember who I was any more.

Sometimes I sit by the fountain in the mall with my charcoal and sketchbook, trying to catch in ten seconds the sling of a belly over a belt or the wobbly scallop of body rolls. I have to go to the mall to find fat people to draw because they don't seem to want to model. Day after day in figure-drawing class, I drew skinny young people with straight-line bodies—bony hips, meatless thighs, hardly a bump at the biceps. If those models only knew how boring I thought their bodies were—until the day we got a blonde woman with breasts that actually shook, a belly that pushed out from her ribs and thighs that showed no muscles. She glided through the quick poses, holding her chest as still as possible, but it was hard to pay attention to the movement I was supposed to be drawing. The curves and volume of her gold-lit body, the kind of figure Rubens would have molded with red and orange and yellow, made motion, and bones, irrelevant. She arranged herself on a faded old easy chair for the long pose. Cellulite dimpled the thigh that sagged over the chair seat, her belly flopped on her hip, and a shoulder without a clavicle blended into her swelled upper arm. She was big and loose, and I couldn't draw any part of her with a straight line. I followed her curves with my eyes and arm and felt my charcoal sinking into her flesh. I shaded her thighs and hips and shoulders; as I moved from dark to light, the energy of her mass softened the touch of my hand on the drawing. I looked at the paper and found lines that I didn't know I could draw—the dangle of her arm over the chair seat, the droopy fullness of her breast. The lines connected me with her, made me see and feel her solid and beautiful whole.

Fat people at the mall get nervous when they see me drawing them, but I don't think they know that on paper they're not fat. On paper, where I take away their three dimensions and put them into two, they're powerful, not flabby; fascinating, not shocking; more human than any unpadded bones could ever be. Black and white and shades of gray strip away suffering, take the flesh out of flesh, make bigness bounty. Sometimes I look at my own fat and hope that someday someone will draw me.

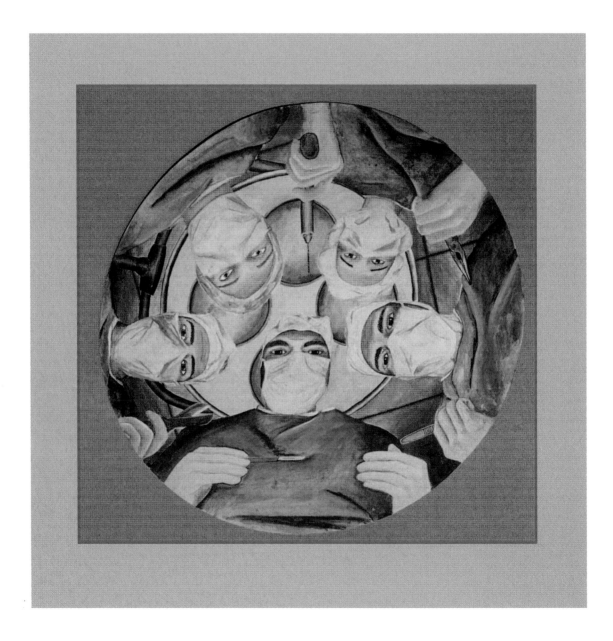

WHAT I KNOW FROM NOSES

Anndee Hochman

FROM THE TIME I WAS EIGHT YEARS OLD, I UNDERSTOOD THAT NOSES, EVEN IF THEY WERE NOT BROKEN, COULD BE MENDED. My aunt had had a nose job, and she wasn't shy about it. I sat next to her on the couch while we paged through old photo albums. "There I am with my old nose," she sometimes said, as if the old nose were a childhood friend who had moved away.

I never asked my aunt why she had her nose fixed. The question seemed too obvious. The old one was too big and too bumpy. Who would pick a bumpy nose, a Jewish nose, if she had the choice? My aunt's new nose looked normal—not too wide or too thin, not too flared at the nostrils or uneven at the bridge. Not a nose anyone would look at twice in a crowded elevator. Which was, I guessed, the idea.

My aunt seemed happy with her new nose. When she smiled, her whole face thrilled—her teeth gleamed and her cheekbones nudged upward, and her nose did not do anything at all. Everyone in the family said she was very photogenic. I thought she was beautiful.

Left: Giles Horton, Anaesthetic or not.

I am in high school, sitting in music class. The wooden chair prods hard against my back; tears burn my eyes. I am fifteen. At just under five feet, I've grown as tall as I'm going to get, and my body has changed. In the sixth grade, my straight dark hair crinkled first into waves, then wiry, unruly kinks. I'm no longer underweight. And my nose, true to family form, has developed a bump.

I look at photographs from before I grew, before my face turned traitor, and I want to cry. I rub my finger down the length of my nose. It feels huge where the bone rises. I think it is growing. At home, with the bathroom door locked, I turn sideways in front of the mirror and hold one hand over my nose, imagining how much better I'd look if it fell straight and smooth from bridge to tip.

On buses, in department stores, at the movies, I see noses attached to people. I judge the noses—too big, too snubbed, better than mine, worse than mine. I hardly see any that are worse than mine.

I am determined not to cry in music class. But Bob Fitzsimmons has just called me "suicide slope." Not for the first time. Across the room, he is snickering about my nose, his shoulders twitching as he whispers to the boy sitting next to him. Bob Fitzsimmons has too many freckles, he wears ugly clothes, and I hate him. I hate my nose.

After dinner that night, I sob to my mother. Everyone thinks I'm ugly, I tell her. I want a new nose. I want this one fixed. She hugs me tightly. OK, she says, OK. We'll go see some doctors.

I started my junior year in high school with crisp looseleaf binders, several medium-point black Bic pens, and a new nose. The operation wasn't so bad. At one point I started to surface out of the anesthesia and felt someone tapping in the middle of my face. It didn't hurt; it just felt annoying, like a headache you wish would go away.

For a week, I wore a bandage and didn't leave the house; for the rest of the summer, I had to be careful not to let my nose get sunburned. In August my father took a picture of me standing on our front walk. I had let my hair grow long since school let out; I wore a wide-brimmed straw hat and a white sundress. I angled my head at the camera, letting my nose show, and smiled widely. It was the first photograph of myself I remember liking.

Back at school, my life was much the same as the year before. I got A's in my classes, wrote for the newspaper, woke up at 6:15 every morning so I could spend forty-five minutes blow-drying the curls out of my hair. But inside myself, I felt changed.

My boyfriend told me, in cramped printing on a sheepishly sweet card, that he thought I was pretty. I believed him. When I acted in school plays, I didn't hesitate to turn my profile to the audience. And on buses, eventually, I stopped noticing the noses first.

More than a decade later, I'm still just barely five feet tall and weigh the same as I did at fifteen. In college I quit wrestling my hair straight; now I wash it and let it dry in random curls. I rarely use makeup. In the summer, I shave my legs from the knees down. "My concession to polite society," I tell my mother.

Sometimes I stand in line at Safeway, turning the glossy pages of women's magazines. Hair dyes, depilatories, plastic surgeries, polymer fingernails, page after page of creams and blushes and eyeliners and lip glosses, page after page of implicit promises: Use this and you'll be beautiful, slender, deliriously happy. These women don't look like me; they don't look like anyone I've ever met. I stuff the magazines back in their racks and pay for my tofu, my spinach, my mineral water. I feel pleased that I'm not buying nail polish.

As a matter of principle, I declare I will never dye gray out of my hair, wear blue contact lenses on my brown eyes, or buy clothes that feel terrible just because they're in style. I tell myself that wearing one's natural face out in the world is not only an honest act, but a political one.

And for all these fourteen years I have carried a secret glitch in my principles, a bump as big as an old nose.

Unlike my aunt, I never talked about my nose job once I left high school. Not even my lovers knew. If friends came to visit at my parents' house, I made sure they saw only baby pictures with my cute snub of a nose, not the telltale "before" photos of adolescence.

It wasn't the nose itself that bothered me so much as the raw spot in my consciousness. I didn't want to remember a time of cringing at nose jokes and hiding my profile from my father's camera. I didn't want to recall how I stung with embarrassment and shame and the desperate hunger to look "right."

As I grew older, questions and arguments haunted my decision. Who says a bumpy nose is bad? Who cares what people think? Why is it mostly Jewish girls who get their noses fixed, Jewish noses that poke across the boundaries of what is considered beautiful? If you change a part of your physical self permanently, what happens to the intangible parts; does your psyche also shift to fit the new shape?

Sometimes, in the bathroom with the door locked, I looked in the mirror and cupped my hand against my nose, making a space where the bump used to be. I wondered then what I had lost when I asked the surgeon to scrape my bone down to smooth—and how I could get it back.

In the last few years, I have begun to tell friends about my nose. The whole story comes back to me vividly: the burn I felt at fifteen, wanting so badly to be pretty. The relief afterward, then all the years of embarrassed, guilty silence. And this realization: that when I stopped seeing noses everywhere I turned, my vision gained room for other things—my whole self, people around me, the desires that webbed us together.

Maybe I would have shed that self-consciousness anyway, slipped gradually out of it and into adulthood. Maybe if I hadn't had a nose job, I would be the same person I am now, just with a rougher profile. I don't believe that chromosomes drive destiny. But I do know that removing the bump on my nose somehow helped me to see past it.

If I ever have a daughter, and her nose takes after mine, and it makes her miserable, I'm not sure what I will tell her. Maybe I'll discuss sexist codes of attractiveness and tell her she's gorgeous just as she is. Maybe I'll hold her tightly and say, OK, let's go talk to some doctors.

I would want my daughter to know this: On the subject of women and beauty, it is the rules, not our bodies, that need repair. But even as I talk, I will remember myself at fifteen—how much, how fervently I wanted and deserved to feel fixed.

Right: Alfred Stieglitz, *Georgia O'Keeffe.*

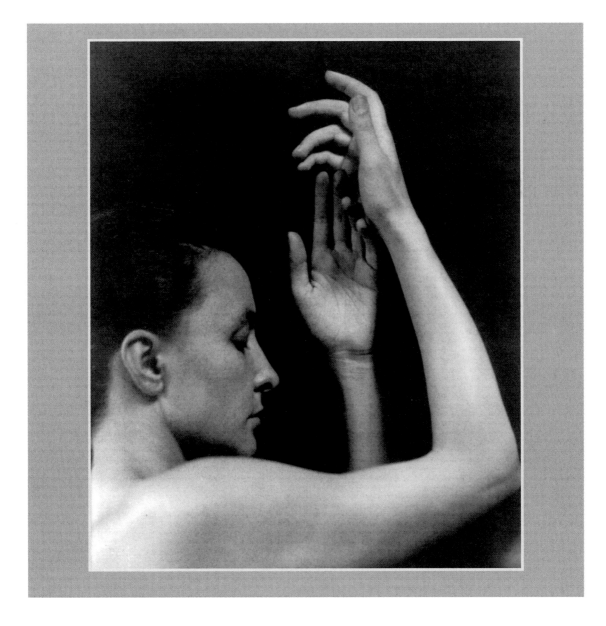

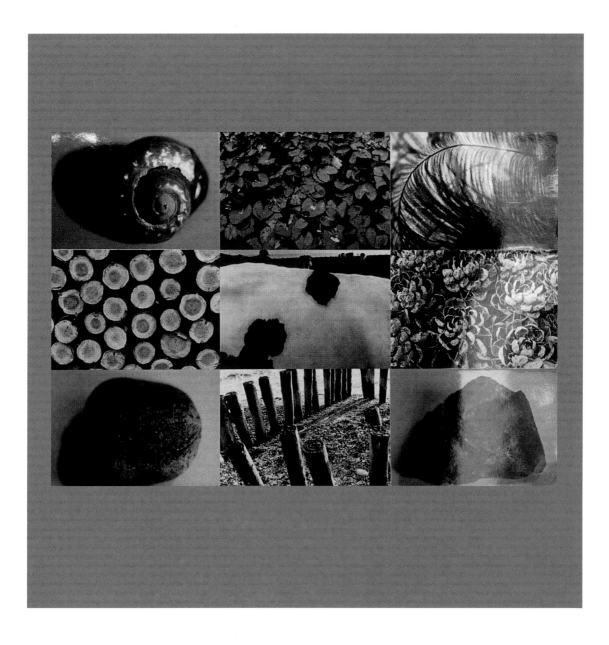

I ACCEPT ALL THE PARTS OF MYSELF

Louise Hay

*Look in the
mirror and say:
"I love
and accept myself
exactly as I am."
What comes up
in your mind?
Notice how you feel.
This may be the
center of your
problem.*

THE BIGGEST PART OF HEALING OR MAKING OURSELVES WHOLE IS TO ACCEPT ALL OF OURSELVES, ALL OF THE MANY PARTS OF ourselves. The times when we did well, and the times when we didn't do so well. The times when we were terrified, and the times when we were loving. The times when we were very foolish and silly, and the times when we were very bright and clever. The times when we had egg on our faces, and the times when we were winners. All of these are parts of ourselves. Most of our problems come from rejecting parts of ourselves—not loving ourselves totally and unconditionally. Let's not look back on our lives with shame. Look at the past as the richness and fullness of Life. Without this richness and fullness we would not be here today. When we accept all of ourselves we become whole and healed.

Left: Sarah Pletts, *Elements.* Both artist and author combine elements to create a new whole.

THE TWELVE
STEPS OF
AMERICAN
RECOVERY
GROUPS

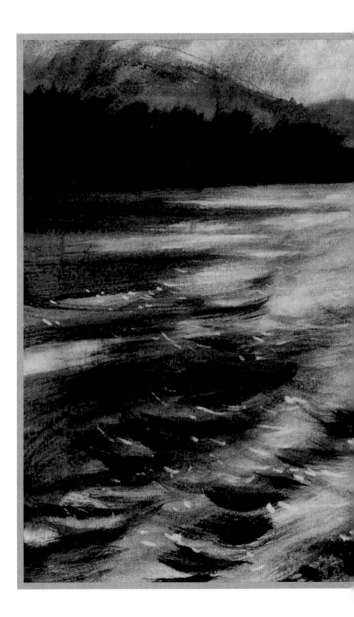

THE AL ANON FAMILY GROUPS ARE A fellowship of relatives and friends of alcoholics who share their experience, strength and hope in order to solve their common problems. We believe alcoholism is a family illness and that changed attitudes can aid recovery.

Al-Anon is not allied with any sect, denomination, political entity, organization or institution; does not engage in any controversy,

Right: Nick Andrew, Holme.
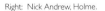

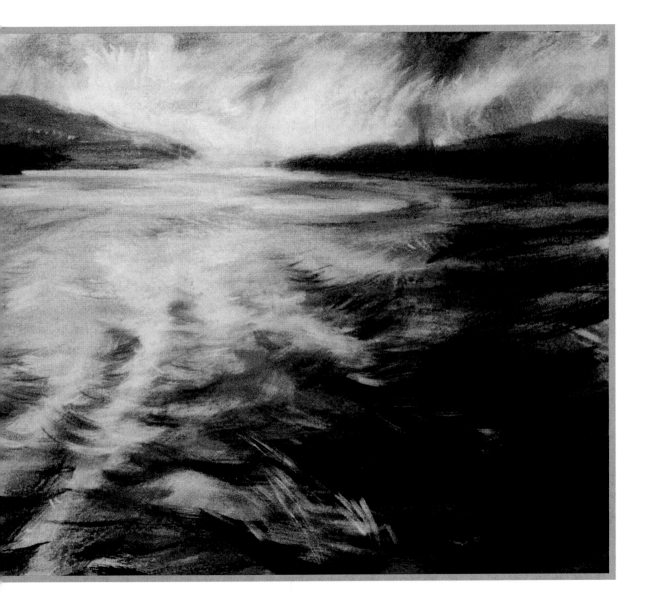

neither endorses nor opposes any cause. There are no dues for membership. Al-Anon is self-supporting through its own voluntary contributions.

Al-Anon has but one purpose: to help families of alcoholics. We do this by practicing the Twelve Steps, by welcoming and giving comfort to families of alcoholics, and by giving understanding and encouragement to the alcoholic.

THE TWELVE STEPS

1. We admitted we were powerless over alcohol-that our lives had become unmanageable.
2. Came to believe that a Power greater than ourselves could restore us to sanity.
3. Made a decision to turn our will and our lives over to the care of God *as we understood Him.*
4. Made a searching and fearless moral inventory of ourselves.
5. Admitted to God, to ourselves and to another human being the exact nature of our wrongs.
6. Were entirely ready to have God remove all these defects of character.
7. Humbly asked Him to remove our shortcomings.
8. Made a list of all persons we had harmed, and became willing to make amends to them all.
9. Made direct amends to such people wherever possible, except when to do so would injure them or others.
10. Continued to take personal inventory and when we were, wrong promptly admitted it.
11. Sought through prayer and meditation to improve our conscious contact with God *as we understood Him,* praying only for knowledge of His will for us and the power to carry that out.
12. Having had a spiritual awakening as the result of these Steps, we tried to carry this message to others, and to practice these principles in all our affairs.

Right: Nick Andrew, *Carpire.*

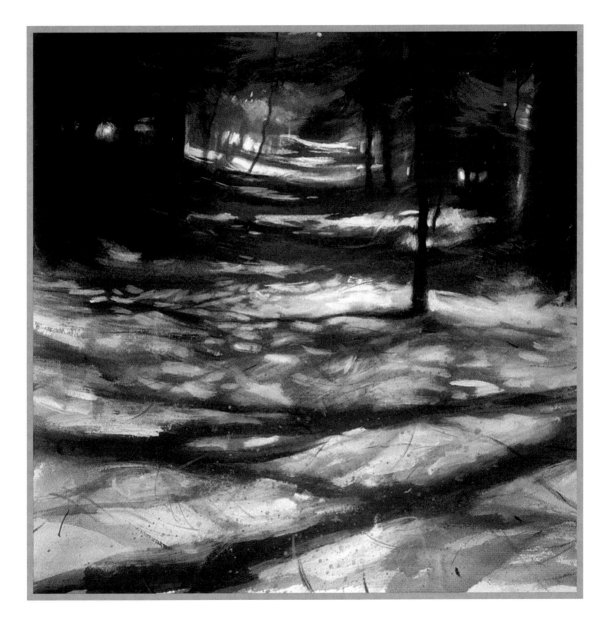

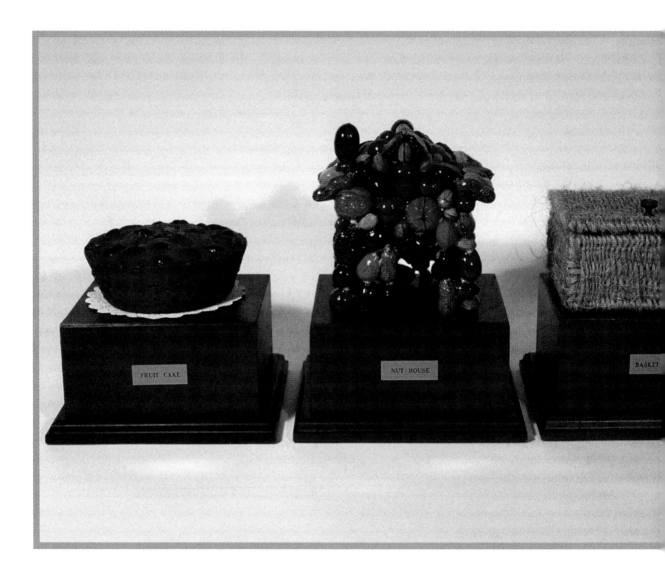

DE-STRESS OR DISTRESS?

Madeleine Begun Kane

ARE YOU STRESSED OUT? A QUIVERING BLOB OF NERVES? ARE YOUR MUSCLES LODGED IN A permanent clench? Here's what not to do:

1. Lie down on the floor with your knees bent and pointed upward. Close your eyes, take a deep breath, and exhale slowly. Take another deep breath. Wonder if that smell is gas.

2. Concentrate on your breathing, on releasing that stale, toxic, virulent energy trapped inside you. Feel your body begin to relax. Sense the tension seeping out of your shoulders and toes, your life force beginning to renew. Jump up to check the stove.

Left: Adrienne Waltking, *Mental Label Series: The Fruit Cake, Nut House and Basket Case.* Both art and story show a sense of humor about health issues which are normally treated with a far more serious tone.

3. Resume the position. Resume breathing. Become obsessed by cobwebs on the ceiling.

4. Decide to play a relaxation tape. Your choices are "healing" harps, ocean waves, and whales. Wonder which best suits your persona. Go with the whales.

5. Lie down a third time, notice ceiling, slam eyelids shut. Breathe deeply, welcoming the return of your vital juices. I.n.h.a.l.e. . . t.w.o. . . t.h.r.e.e. . . fo.u.r. . . E.x.h.a.l.e. . . t.w.o. . . t.h.r.e.e. . . fo.u.r. Savor the rise and fall of your abdomen. Decide whale sounds are weird.

6. Switch to ocean waves and return to floor. Wonder how many calories you've burned since you started to relax.

7. Listen to the primal sounds of the sea. Imagine yourself one with the ocean, gently floating, bobbing, drifting away from your troubles, away from the shore, floating away from. . . Oh my god you're drowning, you can't breathe, you hear chimes. Could you be nearing heaven? No. A Jehovah's Witness is at the door.

8. Decide what you really need is some herbal tea and aroma-therapy. You're all out, so you drive down town to CHAKRAS "R" US.

9. Relish the shop's soothing ambience; crystals everywhere, scented candles and incense, the mellifluous sounds of sitar and flute. Take a slow, deep breath and cherish the knowledge that all is well with the world. Learn you're allergic to patchouli.

10. Fill cart with eucalyptus oil, semi-wild ginseng, organic rice cakes, anti-radiation shields, a do-it-yourself acupuncture kit, and a copy of the best-selling "Bliss Is From Solitude, Stress Is From Men." While your purchases are being processed, grab a "Couple's Massager," just in case.

11. On your way out, collide with a shopping cart piled high with meditation tapes. Exchange choice words with "mellow" New Ager.

12. Return home, light lemon-scented candles, and start a John Tesh CD. Brew camomile tea. Scald tongue with tea.

13. Peruse course catalogue from Holistic Vital Force Renewal and Emerging Spiritual Consciousness Learning and Humanistic Wellness Center.

14. Try to decide which course would be more helpful—Awakening Your True Transformational Self Within Through Toe-Nail Therapy and Micro-Cranial Stimulation? Self-Care, Self-Help, Self-Awareness, Self-Visualization And The Angelic I? Decide to enroll in The Tao Of Conga Drumming On The Far Side Of Ecstasy. . . until you see the price.

15. Conclude that what you really need is a mantra. Something like:
    "NOOOOOOOOOOOOMMMMMMOOOOOOOOOOOOOOOOOOORE NEW AGE."

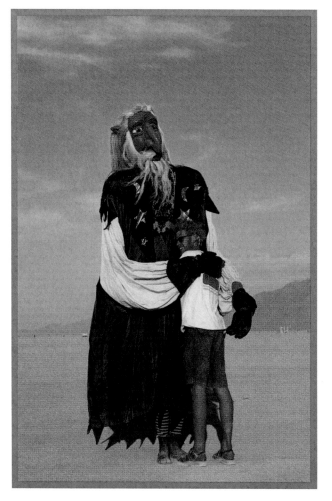

THANK YOU, M'AM

Langston Hughes

S HE WAS A LARGE WOMAN WITH A large purse that had everything in it but a hammer and nails. It had a long strap, and she carried it slung across her shoulder. It was about eleven o'clock at night, dark, and she was walking alone, when a boy ran up behind her and tried to snatch her purse. The strap broke with the sudden single tug the boy gave it from behind. But the boy's weight and the weight of the purse

Left: Burning Man 2001, Photography by Tony Pletts. Meeting someone bigger than oneself—in the art physically and in the story psychologically—has a healing effect on us.

combined caused him to lose his balance. Instead of taking off full blast as he had hoped, the boy fell on his back on the sidewalk and his legs flew up. The large woman simply turned around and kicked him right square in his blue-jeaned sitter. Then she reached down, picked the boy up by his shirt front, and shook him until his teeth rattled.

After that the woman said, "Pick up my pocketbook, boy, and give it here."

She still held him tightly. But she bent down enough to permit him to stoop and pick up her purse. Then she said, "Now ain't you ashamed of yourself?"

Firmly gripped by his shirt front, the boy said, "Yes'm."

The woman said, "What did you want to do it for?"

The boy said, "I didn't aim to."

She said, "You a lie!"

By that time two or three people passed, stopped, turned to look, and some stood watching.

"If I turn you loose, will you run?" asked the woman.

"Yes'm," said the boy.

"Then I won't turn you loose," said the woman. She did not release him.

"Lady, I'm sorry," whispered the boy.

"Um-hum! Your face is dirty. I got a great mind to wash your face for you. Ain't you got nobody home to tell you to wash your face?"

"No'm," said the boy.

"Then it will get washed this evening," said the large woman, starting up the street, dragging the frightened boy behind her.

He looked as if he were fourteen or fifteen, frail and willow-wild, in tennis shoes and blue jeans.

The woman said, "You ought to be my son. I would teach you right from wrong. Least I can do right now is to wash your face. Are you hungry?"

"No'm," said the being-dragged boy. "I just want you to turn me loose."

"Was I bothering *you* when I turned that corner?" asked the woman.

"No'm."

"But you put yourself in contact with *me*," said the woman. "If you think that that contact is not going to last awhile, you got another thought coming. When I get through with you, sir, you are going to remember

Mrs. Luella Bates Washington Jones."

Sweat popped out on the boy's face and he began to struggle. Mrs. Jones stopped, jerked him around in front of her, put a half nelson about his neck, and continued to drag him up the street. When she got to her door, she dragged the boy inside, down a hall, and into a large kitchenette-furnished room at the rear of the house. She switched on the light and left the door open. The boy could hear other roomers laughing and talking in the large house. Some of their doors were open, too, so he knew he and the woman were not alone. The woman still had him by the neck in the middle of her room.

She said, "What is your name?"

"Roger," answered the boy.

"Then, Roger, you go to that sink and wash your face," said the woman, whereupon she turned him loose—at last. Roger looked at the door—looked at the woman-looked at the door—*and went to the sink.*

"Let the water run until it gets warm," she said. "Here's a clean towel."

"You gonna take me to jail?" asked the boy, bending over the sink.

"Not with that face, I would not take you nowhere," said the woman. "Here I am trying to get home to cook me a bite to eat, and you snatch my pocketbook! Maybe you ain't been to your supper either, late as it be. Have you?"

"There's nobody home at my house," said the boy.

"Then we'll eat," said the woman. "I believe you're hungry—or been hungry—to try to snatch my pocketbook!"

"I want a pair of blue suede shoes," said the boy.

"Well, you didn't have to snatch *my* pocketbook to get some suede shoes," said Mrs. Luella Bates Washington Jones. "You could of asked me."

"M'am?"

The water dripping from his face, the boy looked at her. There was a long pause. A very long pause. After he had dried his face, and not knowing what else to do, dried it again, the boy turned around, wondering what next. The door was open. He could make a dash for it down the hall. He could run, run, run, *run!*

The woman was sitting on the daybed. After a while she said, "I were young once and I wanted things I could not get."

There was another long pause. The boy's mouth opened. Then he frowned, not knowing he frowned.

The woman said, "Um-hum! You thought I was going to say *but*, didn't you? You thought I was going to say, *but I didn't snatch people's pocketbooks.* Well, I wasn't going to say that." Pause. Silence. "I have done things, too, which I would not tell you, son—neither tell God, if He didn't already know. Everybody's got something in common. So you set down while I fix us something to eat. You might run that comb through your hair so you will look presentable."

In another corner of the room behind a screen was a gas plate and an icebox. Mrs. Jones got up and went behind the screen. The woman did not watch the boy to see if he was going to run now, nor did she watch her purse, which she left behind her on the daybed. But the boy took care to sit on the far side of the room, away from the purse, where he thought she could easily see him out of the corner of her eye if she wanted to. He did not trust the woman *not* to trust him. And he did not want to be mistrusted now.

"Do you need somebody to go to the store," asked the boy, maybe to get some milk or something?"

"Don't believe I do," said the woman, "unless you just want sweet milk yourself. I was going to make cocoa out of this canned milk I got here."

"That will be fine," said the boy.

She heated some lima beans and ham she had in the icebox, made the cocoa, and set the table. The woman did not ask the boy anything about where he lived, or his folks, or anything else that would embarrass him. Instead, as they ate, she told him about her job in a hotel beauty shop that stayed open late, what the work was how like and how all kinds of women came in and out, blonds, redheads, and Spanish. Then she cut him a half of her ten-cent cake.

"Eat some more, son," she said.

When they were finished eating, she got up and said, "Now here, take this ten dollars and buy yourself some blue suede shoes. And next time, do not make the mistake of latching onto *my* pocketbook *nor nobody else's*—because shoes got by devilish ways will burn your feet. I got to get my rest now. But from here on in, son, I hope you will behave yourself."

She led him down the hall to the front door and opened it. "Good night! Behave yourself, boy!" she said, looking out into the street as he went down the steps.

The boy wanted to say something other than, "Thank you, M'am," to Mrs. Luella Bates Washington Jones, but although his lips moved, he couldn't even say that as he turned at the foot of the barren stoop and looked up at the large woman in the door. Then she shut the door.

T H E   L E A F   S H A P E   R E M A I N S

John Fox

WHEN I WAS EIGHTEEN MY RIGHT LEG WAS AMPUTATED JUST BELOW MY KNEE. I HAD NUMEROUS SURGERIES SINCE the age of five to save a deformed leg from the ongoing ravages of a genetic disorder called neurofibromotosis, and before the amputation I had spent that year as a university freshman in Boston struggling with a leg I could barely walk on. The poems I wrote during that time of emotional distress and physical pain made an enormous difference to me.

My work as a poetry therapist and teacher is deeply influenced by that particular experience. Yet that year of suffering wasn't when my enchantment with poetry began. Something I experienced much earlier in my life fed the deepest root of my instincts as a writer, the root that keeps me growing. It was the pure desire to create, to make. It preceded everything. I was thirteen years old, watching a girl skate at a rink in Shaker Heights, Ohio, and I decided to write my first poem—a torrent of words related to beauty, attraction and risk. I wanted my words to skate on the page and I sensed so much joy as I wrote.

I made books of poems in my adolescence and gave them away to people, mostly women: a girlfriend whose love I wanted to win, a teacher who valued my perceptions. I wrote and I wrote, and looking back, it's clear I was giving voice to, as John Keats understood, my heart's affections and the truth of the imagination.

This deeply rooted connection to something beautiful and to the range of feelings surging within me, gave me a sense of my own internal richness and of life's essential mysteries. Writing poetry became a direct link to the unknown, and it felt real. Nothing else would be more important as I entered the country of grief.

Although I walked on a prosthesis within a month after the amputation (I even played on a softball team of former high school friends that summer—a friend ran for me as I stood up to hit), the pain remained intense. For years, doctors prescribed strong pain relievers but to no avail. Nothing alleviated the pain that burned like streamers of fire in my now-absent leg.

Someone who experiences the death of or separation from a loved one may imagine that person smiling or walking around a corner or hear their voice say "hello" when answering the phone. What they

Right: Georgia O'Keeffe, *Yellow Hickory Leaves with Daisy.*

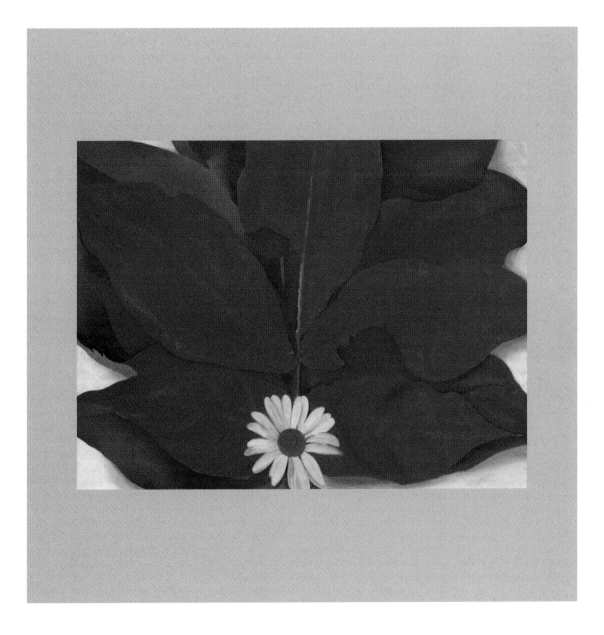

discover is that sunlight has hit upon a stranger's face at a certain angle leaving a shadow of hope, or that a familiar vocal inflection is only an unknown person's wrong number. Similarly, phantom pain is an exquisite metaphor for loss. What you lose never really goes away.

After I lost my leg, I wanted to get beyond the physical and emotional pain, but my sense of shame was deeply entrenched and the unexpected intensity of the phantom pain unsettled me. When I returned to school the following autumn, I sought counseling, meditated at a Buddhist center in Cambridge, and attended a poetry workshop with George Starbuck. They were all helpful, but I was still unable to wholly confront my deepest grief and fear.

Injuring my stump finally provided the circumstance that led to a turning point in my writing and in my life. Because of a relatively small contusion, I could not wear the prosthesis, and for two or three days I holed up in my dorm room trying to gather the courage to venture out onto Commonwealth Avenue and into my classrooms—with the right leg of my pants pinned up. I couldn't do it. I couldn't make a move out of my room. But I did write a poem of aching truth, of deep longing.

Even to This

What my thoughts have troubled about
all through the night after night!

It's so very scary
　　　sometimes
　I feel
　　　　　would rather. . . .

what's the worst that could happen?
because it just hurts too much

or having had enough of my own self-hatred
against myself, lonely is

nowhere else to go—
time to stop feeling sorry
for myself,

time to open my heart
even to this
and call to God.

What does one do with grief? Poetry can enter into the severed places in life that explanations and reason do not touch. The open nature of the blank page allows you to experiment with releasing that hurt. Poems of grief can offer a diamond-like truth, an insight-surprise that is sheer gift. "Hard won" is often the nature of these poems. Yet they neither exhaust me nor outgrow their usefulness; rather, they continue to teach generously over time. Sometimes I come in contact with an essential joy behind the pain. Writing poems that reveal this unexpected light feels like receiving grace. And very often such poems seem to write themselves.

I did not know what my next step would be until I wrote the above poem. My experience was only of writing, like throwing fragments of my troubled thoughts onto the page. I let my thoughts appear in seemingly unconnected pieces and wrote the shape of my hurt. In my willingness to show and say what I feared, I discovered that my next step was not to get rid of the pain but to acknowledge it. The pain of losing my leg was like a guest I hadn't invited but who nonetheless had to be received.

Accepting the loss of my leg seemed more possible—and more transformational—after writing this poem. I began to put my attention and care into acknowledging my loss, rather than medicating myself and dulling the pain. My poem told me: making a place in my heart for the loss of my leg could help. If I didn't do this, something else less healthy would move into that space of loss and claim my life energy.

My grief about the loss, my fear of the future, the self-hatred and loneliness woven into my turbulent feelings and thoughts—all of these asked not for painkillers but for opening—for opening "even to this." There was nothing else for me to do. First I had to tell myself there was "nowhere else to go." If I refused to accept my loss, I would be trapped by something even more debilitating than physical pain: self-pity. Self-pity had no point, no message. Its only function was to keep my heart tightly contracted and my soul hopeless. Feeling sorry for myself allowed no room for seeing what is—or for letting God into my life.

The more I looked at my poem, I realized that a deep relationship existed between accepting what is and help from God. Coming to an emotional awareness of what I needed made my last four words "and call to God" feel true, unexpected, deeply felt, natural. I experienced a powerful sense of breaking through—without disowning myself. Writing made this possible!

After writing the poem, I tried healing exercises in place of painkillers. I visualized velvety rose-petals floating down over my stump. Using this vibrant image eased the pain considerably and opened my heart to the reality of my loss. I did this with actual rose petals. How beautiful to see my stump strewn not with hot embers of rejection and self-pity but the velvet petals of letting go.

My experience at thirteen of being inspired by a skater—by a grace that opened my life to poetry—also taught me more than I knew at the time about the courage to both live and to write. Thinking back on that initial vision of the skater, I wrote this poem in 1999:

Poetry

It skates boldly onto
the page, tips one vulnerable foot
back and forth slowly, till finally
the edge of a toe
cuts a simple, sharp line
through the world's cold resistance
and with that plain courage, a statement of intention begins;
and you can't turn back any longer
from the weight of feeling and letting go
into the flow that follows.
Poetry is a choice to feel it all,
not all at once but gradually to sink down
within ourselves, to give what fear
we hold behind our knees
to gravity and grace,
to discover what makes
our whole world turn;
the place our necessary weight
lifts to lightened joy.

Right: Alfred Stieglitz, *Equivalent.*

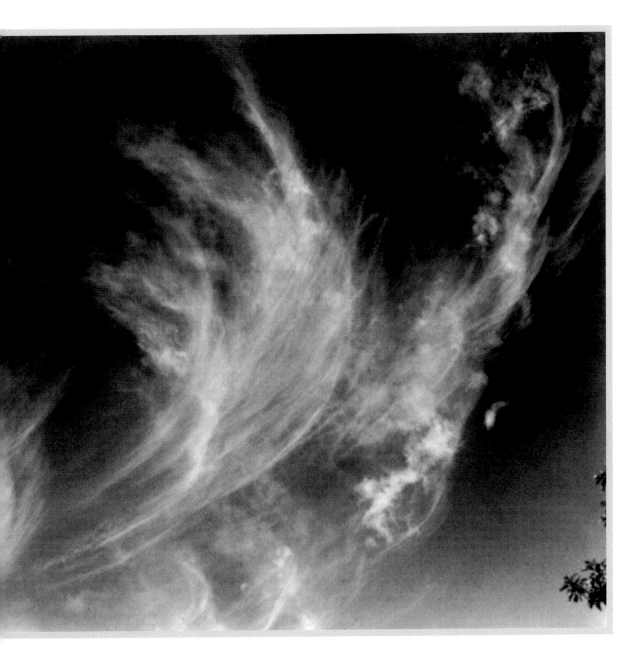

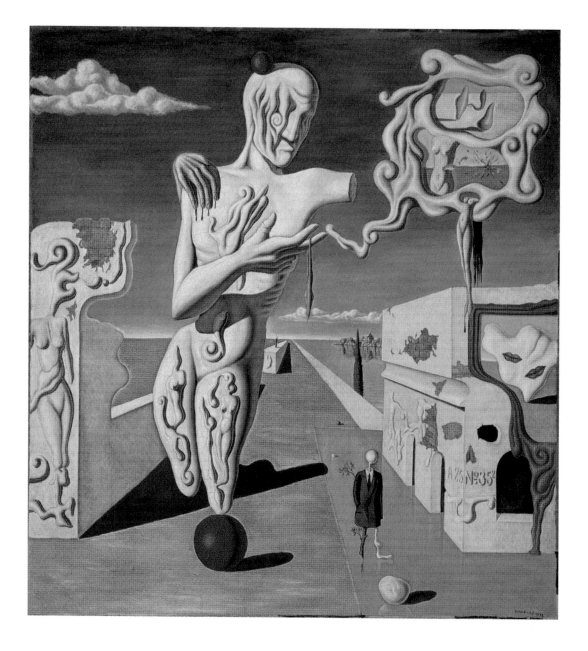

LISTENING TO PROZAC

Peter D. Kramer

MY FIRST EXPERIENCE WITH PROZAC INVOLVED A WOMAN I WORKED WITH ONLY AROUND ISSUES OF MEDICATION. A psychologist with whom I collaborate had called to say she was treating a patient who had accomplished remarkable things in adult life despite an especially grim childhood; now, in her early thirties, the patient had become clinically depressed. Would I see her in consultation? My colleague summarized the woman's history, and I learned more when Tess arrived at my office.

Tess was the eldest of ten children born to a passive mother and an alcoholic father in the poorest public-housing project in our city. She was abused in childhood in the concrete physical and sexual senses which everyone understands as abuse. When Tess was twelve, her father died, and her mother entered a clinical depression from which she had never recovered. Tess—one of those inexplicably resilient children who flourish without any apparent source of sustenance—took over the family. She managed to remain in school herself and in time to steer all nine siblings into stable jobs and marriages.

Her own marriage was less successful. At seventeen, she married an older man, in part to provide a base outside the projects for her younger brothers and sisters, whom she immediately took in. She never went to the movies alone with her husband; the children came along. The weight of the family was always on her shoulders. The husband was alcoholic, and abusive when drunk. Tess struggled to help him stop drinking, but to no avail. The marriage soon became loveless. It collapsed once the children—Tess's siblings—were grown and one of its central purposes had disappeared.

Meanwhile, Tess had made a business career out of her skills at driving, inspiring, and nurturing others. She achieved a reputation as an administrator capable of turning around struggling companies by addressing issues of organization and employee morale, and she rose to a high level in a large corporation. She

Left: Angel Plannells, *Midday Sorrow.*

still cared for her mother, and she kept one foot in the projects, sitting on the school committee, working with the health clinics, investing personal effort in the lives of individuals who mostly would disappoint her.

It is hard to overstate how remarkable I found the story of Tess's success. I had an image of her beginnings. The concrete apartment in which she cared for her younger brothers and sisters was recently destroyed with great fanfare on local television. Years earlier, my work as head of a hospital clinic had led me to visit that building. From the start, it must have been a vertical prison, a place where to survive at all could be counted as high ambition. To succeed as Tess had—and without a stable family to guide or support her—was almost beyond imagining.

That her personal life was unhappy should not have been surprising. Tess stumbled from one prolonged affair with an abusive married man to another. As these degrading relationships ended, she would suffer severe demoralization. The current episode had lasted months, and, despite a psychotherapy in which Tess willingly faced the difficult aspects of her life, she was now becoming progressively less energetic and more unhappy. It was this condition I hoped to treat, in order to spare Tess the chronic and unremitting depression that had taken hold in her mother when she was Tess's age . . .

It was the mother's illness that drove me forward. Tess had struggled too long for me to allow her, through any laxness of my own, to slide into the chronic depression that had engulfed her mother.

Depression is a relapsing and recurring illness. The key to treatment is thoroughness. If a patient can put together a substantial period of doing perfectly well—five months, some experts say; six or even twelve, say others—the odds are good for sustained remission. But to limp along just somewhat improved, "better but not well," is dangerous. The partly recovered patient will likely relapse as soon as you stop the therapy, as soon as you taper the drug. And the longer someone remains depressed, the more likely it is that depression will continue or return . . .

I tried a dose of imipramine, but Tess began to experience side effects—dry mouth, daytime tiredness, further weight gain—so we switched to similar medications in hopes of finding one that would allow her to tolerate a higher dose. Tess changed little.

And then Prozac was released by the Food and Drug Administration. I prescribed it for Tess, for entirely conventional reasons—to terminate her depression more thoroughly, to return her to her "premorbid self." My goal was not to transform Tess but to restore her.

But medications do not always behave as we expect them to.

Two weeks after starting Prozac, Tess appeared at the office to say she was no longer feeling weary. In retrospect, she said, she had been depleted of energy for as long as she could remember, had almost not known what it was to feel rested and hopeful. She had been depressed, it now seemed to her, her whole life. She was astonished at the sensation of being free of depression.

She looked different, at once more relaxed and energetic—more available—than I had seen her, as if the person hinted at in her eyes had taken over. She laughed more frequently, and the quality of her laughter was different, no longer measured but lively, even teasing.

With this new demeanor came a new social life, one that did not unfold slowly, as a result of a struggle to integrate disparate parts of the self, but seemed, rather, to appear instantly and full-blown.

"Three dates a weekend," Tess told me. "I must be wearing a sign on my forehead!"

Within weeks of starting Prozac, Tess settled into a satisfying dating routine with men. She had missed out on dating in her teens and twenties. Now she reveled in the attention she received. She seemed even to enjoy the trial-and-error process of learning contemporary courtship rituals, gauging norms for sexual involvement, weighing the import of men's professed infatuation with her.

I had never seen a patient's social life reshaped so rapidly and dramatically. Low self-worth, competitiveness, jealousy, poor interpersonal skills, shyness, fear of intimacy—the usual causes of social awkwardness—are so deeply ingrained and so difficult to influence that ordinarily change comes gradually if at all. But Tess blossomed all at once.

. . . depression is not the soul's annihilation; men and women who have recovered from the disease—and they are countless—bear witness to what is probably its only saving grace: it is conquerable. For those who have dwelt in depression's dark wood, and known its inexplicable agony, their return from the abyss is not unlike the ascent of the poet, trudging upward and upward out of hell's black depths and at last emerging into what he saw as "the shining world." There, whoever has been restored to health has almost always been restored to the capacity for serenity and joy, and this may be indemnity enough for having endured the despair beyond despair.

—William Styron

"People on the sidewalk ask me for directions!" she said. They never had before.

The circle of Tess's women friends changed. Some friends left, she said, because they had been able to relate to her only through her depression. Besides, she now had less tolerance for them. "Have you ever been to a party where other people are drunk or high and you are stone-sober? Their behavior annoys you, you can't understand it. It seems juvenile and self-centered. That's how I feel around some of my old friends. It is as if they are under the influence of a harmful chemical and I am all right—as if I had been in a drugged state all those years and now I am clearheaded."

The change went further: "I can no longer understand how they tolerate the men they are with." She could scarcely acknowledge that she had once thrown herself into the same sorts of self-destructive relationships. "I never think about Jim," she said. And in the consulting room his name no longer had the power to elicit tears.

This last change struck me as most remarkable of all. When a patient displays any sign of masochism, and I think it is fair to call Tess's relationship with Jim masochistic, psychiatrists anticipate a protracted psychotherapy. It is rarely easy to help a socially self-destructive patient abandon humiliating relationships and take on new ones that accord with a healthy sense of self-worth. But once Tess felt better, once the weariness lifted and optimism became possible, the masochism just withered away, and she seemed to have every social skill she needed.

Tess's work, too, became more satisfying. She responded without defensiveness in the face of adamant union leaders, felt stable enough insider herself to evaluate their complaints critically. She said the medication had lent her surety of judgment; she no longer tortured herself over whether she was being too demanding or too lenient . . . . Whether the conflicts were real or illusory, the problem disappeared when the medication took effect. "It makes me confident," Tess said, a claim I since have heard from dozens of patients, none of whom had been given a hint that this medication, or any medication, could do any such thing.

Tess's management style changed. She was less conciliatory, firmer, unafraid of confrontation. As the troubled company settled down, Tess was given a substantial pay raise, a sign that others noticed her new effectiveness. . . .

There is no unhappy ending to this story. It is like one of those Elizabethan dramas—Marlowe's *Tamburlaine*—so foreign to modern audiences because the Wheel of Fortune takes only half a turn: the patient recovers and pays no price for the recovery. Tess did go off medication, after about nine months, and she continued to do well. She was, she reported, not quite so sharp of thought, so energetic, so free of care as she had been on the medication, but neither was she driven by guilt and obligation. She was altogether cooler, better controlled, less sensible of the weight of the world than she had been.

After about eight months off medication, Tess told me she was slipping. "I'm not myself," she said. New union negotiations were under way, and she felt she could use the sense of stability, the invulnerability to attack, that Prozac gave her. Here was a dilemma for me. Ought I to provide medication to someone who was not depressed? I could give myself reason enough—construe it that Tess was sliding into relapse, which perhaps she was. In truth, I assumed I would he medicating Tess's chronic condition, call it what you will: heightened awareness of the needs of others, sensitivity to conflict, residual damage to self-esteem—all odd indications for medication. I discussed the dilemma with her, but then I did not hesitate to write the prescription. Who was I to withhold from her the bounties of science? Tess responded again as she had hoped she would, with renewed confidence, self-assurance, and social comfort.

I believe Tess's story contains an unchronicled reason for Prozac's enormous popularity: its ability to alter personality. Here was a patient whose usual method of functioning changed dramatically. She became socially capable, no longer a wallflower but a social butterfly. Where once she had focused on obligations to others. now she was vivacious and fun-loving. Before, she had pined after men; now she dated them, enjoyed them, weighed their faults and virtues. Newly confident, Tess had no need to romanticize or indulge men's shortcomings.

Not all patients on Prozac respond this way. Some are unaffected by the medicine; some merely recover from depression, as they might on any antidepressant. But a few, a substantial minority, are transformed. Like Garrison Keillor's marvelous Powdermilk biscuits, Prozac gives these patients the courage to do what needs to be done.

B E C O M I N G   M E D I C A L L Y   I N T U I T I V E

Caroline Myss

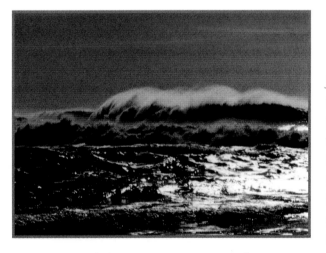

I N THE AUTUMN OF 1982, AFTER ENDING MY career as a newspaper journalist and obtaining a master's degree in theology, I joined forces with two partners to start a book publishing company called Stillpoint. We published books about healing methods that were alternatives to establishment medicine. Despite my business interest in alternative therapies, however, I wasn't the least bit interested in becoming personally involved in them. I had no desire to meet any healers myself. I refused to meditate. I developed an absolute aversion to wind chimes, New Age music, and conversations on the benefits of organic gardening. I smoked while drinking coffee by the gallon, still fashioning myself after an image of a hard-boiled newspaper reporter. I was not at all primed for a mystical experience.

Right: Giles Horton, *Emergence*. Giles shows an older image of himself emerging from a younger one. The story describes the constantly evolving relationship with oneself which is needed for a medical intuitive.

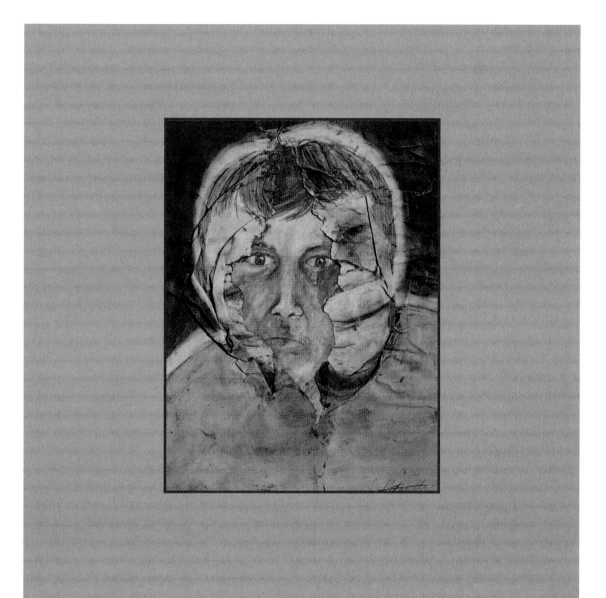

Nonetheless, that same autumn, I gradually recognized that my perceptual abilities had expanded considerably. For instance, a friend would mention that someone he knew was not feeling well, and an insight into the cause of the problem would pop into my head. I was uncannily accurate, and word of it spread through the local community. Soon people were phoning the publishing company to make appointments for an intuitive assessment of their health. By the spring of 1983 I was doing readings for people who were in health crises and life crises of various kinds, from depression to cancer.

To say I was in a fog would be a gross understatement. I was confused and a little scared. I could not figure out how I was getting these impressions. They were, and still are, like impersonal daydreams that start to flow as soon as I receive a person's permission, name, and age. Their impersonality, the nonfeeling sensation of the impressions, is extremely significant because it is my indicator that I am not manufacturing or projecting these impressions. It's like the difference between looking through a stranger's photograph album, in which you have emotional attachments to no one, and looking through your own family's photo album. The impressions are dear but completely unemotional.

Because I also didn't know how accurate my impressions were, after a couple months of consultations I found myself dreading each appointment intensely, feeling each was a high-risk experience. I got through the first six months only by telling myself that using my medical intuition was a bit of a game. I got excited when I made an accurate "hit" because, if nothing else, an accurate hit meant my sanity was intact. Even so, each time I wondered: "Will 'it' work this time? What if no impressions show up? What if I'm wrong about something? What if someone asks me something I can't answer? What if I tell someone she's healthy, only to learn later that she's had a terminal diagnosis? And above all, what's a journalist-theological-student-turned-publisher doing in this borderline occupation in the first place?"

People sometimes ask me where my own healing energy comes from. How in the midst of this pain, this implacable slow crippling, can I encourage myself and other people? My answer is that my healing comes from my bitterness itself, my despair, my terror. It comes from the shadow. I dip down into that muck again and again and am flooded with its healing energy. Despite the renewal and vitality it gives me to face my deepest fears, I don't go willingly when they call. I've been around that wheel a million times: first I feel the despair, but I deny it for a few days; then its tugs become more insistent in proportion to my resistance; and finally it is overwhelming and pulls me down, kicking and screaming all the way. It's clear I am caught, so at last I give up to this reunion with the dark aspect of my adjustment to pain and loss. Immediately the release begins: first peace and then the flood of vitality and healing energy.

—Darlene Cohen

I felt as if I were suddenly responsible for explaining the will of God to dozens of sad, frightened people, without any training. Ironically, the more these folks wanted insight into what God was doing to them, the more I wanted insight into what God was doing to me. The pressure I felt finally resulted in years of migraine headaches.

I wanted to carry on as if my emerging skill were no different from a talent for baking, but I knew better. Having grown up Catholic and studied theology, I was keenly aware that transpersonal abilities lead one inevitably to the monastery—or to the madhouse. Deep in my soul, I knew that I was connecting with something that was essentially sacred, and that knowledge was splitting me in two. On the one hand, I feared that I would become incapacitated, like mystics of old; on the other, I felt destined for a life in which I would be evaluated and judged by believers and skeptics. No matter how I envisioned my future, however, I felt I was headed for misery.

But I was fascinated by my newfound perceptual ability, nonetheless, and was compelled to keep on evaluating people's health. In these early days the impressions I received were mainly of a person's immediate physical health and the related emotional or psychological stress. But I could also *see* the energy surrounding that person's body. I saw it filled with information about that persons history. And I saw that energy as an extension of that person's spirit. I began to realize something I had never been taught in school: that our spirit is very much a part of our daily lives; it embodies our thoughts and emotions, and it records every one of them, from the most mundane to the visionary. Although I had been taught, more or less, that our spirit goes either "up" or "down" after death, depending upon how virtuously we have lived, I now saw that our spirit is more than that. It participates in every second of our lives. It is the conscious force that is life itself.

I carried on with my health readings on a sort of automatic pilot, until one day my ambivalence toward my skill was resolved. I was in the middle of a session with a woman who had cancer. The day was hot, and I was tired. The woman and I sat facing each other in my small office at Stillpoint. I had completed her evaluation and was hesitating for a moment before sharing it with her. I dreaded telling her that the cancer had spread throughout her body. I knew she was going to ask me why this catastrophe had happened to her, and I felt irritated by my responsibility of answering her. Sure enough, as I opened my mouth to speak, she reached over, put her hand on my leg, and asked, "Caroline, I know I have a serious cancer. Can't you tell me why this is happening to me."

My indignation rose to meet the hated question, and I almost snapped, "How would I know?"—when suddenly I was flushed with an energy I had never felt before. It moved through my body, as if it were pushing me aside in order to make use of my vocal cords. I could no longer see the woman in front of me. I felt as if I had been shrunk down to the size of a dime and ordered to "stand watch" from inside my head.

A voice spoke through me to this woman. "Let me walk you back through your life and through each of the relationships of your life," it said. "Let me walk with you through all the fears you've had, and let me show you how those fears controlled you for so long that the energy of life could no longer nurture you."

This "presence" escorted this woman through every detail of her life, and I mean every detail. It recalled the smallest of conversations for her; it recounted moments of great loneliness in which she had wept by herself; it remembered every relationship that had held any meaning for her. This "presence" left the impression that every second of our lives—and every mental, emotional, creative, physical, and even resting activity with which we fill those seconds—is somehow known and recorded. Every judgment we make is noted. Every attitude we hold is a source of positive or negative power for which we are accountable.

I was awestruck by this experience. From the sidelines I began to pray, half out of fear and half out of humility in facing the intimate and ultimate design of the universe. I had always assumed that our prayers are "heard," but I had never been quite sure how. Nor had I figured with my simple human reasoning how any system, even a Divine one, could keep track of everyone's needs, giving requests for healing priority over say, requests for financial assistance. I was unprepared for this sacred spectacle in which every second of life is lovingly held to be of great value.

As I prayed, still only an observer, I asked that this woman remain completely unaware that it was not I who was speaking to her. Since I couldn't have answered her question "Why do I have cancer?" I also couldn't have explained how I knew details about her past. As soon as I released that prayer, I was again looking directly into her face. I found that my hand was on her knee, mirroring her reaching out to me, although I had no recollection of having put it there.

My entire body was trembling and I removed my hand. All she said was, "Thank you so much. I can live with everything now." She paused, then continued, "Even my death doesn't scare me. Everything is just fine."

She left my office and a moment later so did I, in a profoundly shaken state. I walked into a beautiful open field that surrounded Stillpoint and I agreed to cooperate with this intuitive ability, no matter the outcome.

Since that autumn day in 1983 I have worked wholeheartedly as a medical intuitive. This means that I use my intuitive ability to help people understand the emotional, psychological, and spiritual energy that lies at the root of their illness, disease, or life crisis. I can sense the type of illness that has developed, often before the individual is aware of having an illness at all. The people I work with usually are aware, however, that their lives are not in balance and that something is wrong. . . .

For the first two years, I held back much of the information that I sensed. I limited my assistance to helping people interpret the emotional, psychological, and spiritual stresses and factors underlying the development of their illness. I did not discuss specific medical treatments or surgical procedures but instead referred clients to physicians. In 1984, however, I met C. Norman Shealy, M.D., Ph.D. I began intensive training with him in the physical anatomy of the human body. By speaking to and through Norm to patients about their lives and illness, I was able to refine my understanding of the impressions I received. This gave me the comfort zone I needed to permit my skill to mature, although I still do not treat clients and only try to help them interpret the spiritual issues at the root of their emotional or physical crisis. . . .

Being medically intuitive has helped me learn not only about the energy causes of disease but about the challenges we face in healing ourselves. Of great significance to me was the realization that "healing" does not always mean that the physical body recovers from an illness. Healing can also mean that one's spirit has released long-held fears and negative thoughts toward oneself or others. This kind of spiritual release and healing can occur even though one's body may be dying physically.

As a psychotherapist, if I distance myself defensively from the problems my clients bring to me, I force them to carry universal illness while I try to have power over the disease in order to be protected from it. Healing, however, may ask more from the doctor. It may require a willingness to approach the illness as an intimate, as someone interested in the mystery, and as a member of the human community affected by this disease.

—Thomas Moore

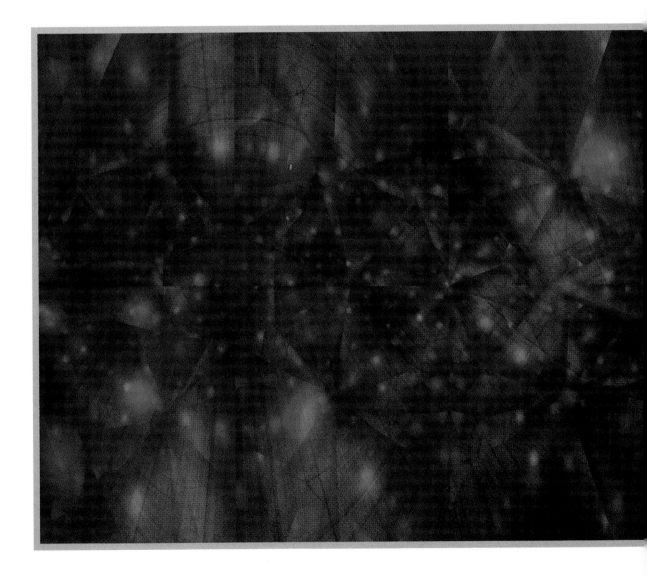

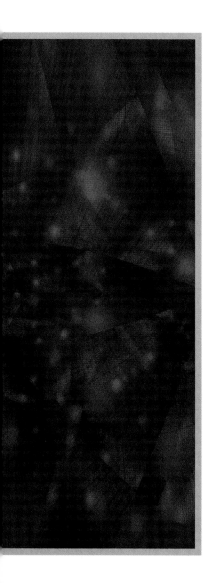

S P I R I T   G U A R D I A N S

Donna Eden

THOUGH ALWAYS UNEXPECTED AND A BIT MYSTICAL, THE APPEARANCE OF spirit guardians occurs often enough in my work that I am forced to come to terms with their sometimes conspicuous presence. Reports of help and guidance from another realm are increasing, and there are sometimes urgent reasons that cause otherworldly help to make itself know. Sometimes it can. More often our conditioning and cultural filters prevent us from becoming conscious of it, but I have many times experienced a presence in a session that provided an important key to the healing process. Here is one of those instances.

I was teaching a class at Palomar College, near San Diego, in the summer of 1981. A woman drew my attention because she never participated in the class, and she generally left just before the sessions ended. She seemed to be in considerable physical pain. I later learned that to attempt this kind of healing without summoning Jesus conflicted with her religious faith, and she felt confused.

Left: Cathryn Chase, *Fireflies.* The subject of the story and of the image share something ethereal.

Eventually, however, the woman asked for an appointment. Betty had suffered with a great deal of pain on her left side since having had polio as a child. Now that she was in her early sixties, her bone structure and musculature weren't carrying her well, and the pain was intensifying, particularly in her left shoulder and hip. She had been to numerous doctors, but none of them had been able to relieve the pain. She had been told, "This is just something you're going to have to learn to live with."

Betty was pleasantly surprised by substantial relief form her pain after our first and then our second sessions. During the third session, I kept having a sense of seeing a red energy in the corner of the room. This didn't compute. I was trying to dismiss it, but it was very demanding. The session was suddenly interrupted. A male, ghostly, almost human figure was standing in that corner. He reminded me of Yul Brynner in *The King and I*, even to the bald head. In a regal way, he commanded: "I am Balasheem. Stand at her shoulders!"

I stood at her shoulders and put my fingers on them. Suddenly it felt like this being stepped into my body. The middle fingers on each hand felt like they had become steel rods that were plugged into her shoulders. I couldn't move them away. Such a strong force of energy pulsed through my body and out of my hands that she began to vibrate, very hard, until it looked as if she were going into convulsions. I was stunned, and I couldn't pull my fingers away. She was moving up and down, up and down, something between vibrating and convulsing, until she fell off the table. Only then did we disconnect.

I rushed to her, thinking, "Oh my God, is she okay?" Betty was sobbing uncontrollably on the floor, and I could do nothing that made her stop. Finally, she said, "Look!" She showed me her increased range of motion and declared that she was having no pain. None whatsoever. It was all gone. She hadn't had full range of motion since prior to her polio, and she hadn't had relief from pain for many years. She began to excitedly wonder aloud if I were "Mary, Mother of Jesus." No other explanation fit for her. Meanwhile, I was saying, "Betty, it wasn't me! It was like a spirit came into me. He called himself Balasheem." "It was Mary and Jesus," she screamed excitedly. "No," I replied, "He said his name was Balasheem, and he looked like Yul Brynner."

She was perplexed. This didn't fit anything she believed, but she could not deny her improved condition. She began telling her church community that Mother Mary was using my body for healings. I was flooded with calls from people wanting me to heal them. At first I was trying to explain, "It wasn't like that; I'm not Mary." Finally, I began to just agree that some divine healing force had apparently come through. I was leaving soon and could not accept any new clients, but I did agree to see Betty one more time.

At that session, she was filled with questions. "Why me?" I didn't have any answers, but I sensed deeply that Balasheem was personally aligned with her, that he was not some generic force of the heavens who was available for everybody. I said that to her, and she responded, "Well, if he comes again, I want to know why he doesn't just talk to me directly!" Suddenly, I could sense him in the room. I said, "Betty, I believe he's here." She said, irritated, "Well, ask him!" I heard the reply, "I have been trying to reach Betty all her life. And now it is imperative that she believe in me." And that was it. He was gone. I didn't know what that meant, that it was *imperative* that she believe in him. She still grumbled, but she was fascinated and felt that regardless of what I wanted to call him—it might have something to do with my own strange spiritual beliefs—she knew that Mother Mary had graced her life.

I left for home. I had no contact with Betty for months. Then, one day as I was walking in the park, I was confronted with the apparition of Balasheem. He just appeared and told me to call Betty. He gave me specific dietary instructions I was to convey to her, having to do with nine vitamins and minerals, the amounts she needed, and what was out of balance. I went straight to the phone and said, "Betty, I saw Balasheem in the park just now, and he told me to call you." I described his dietary suggestions for her. There was a long silence. She finally asked me to repeat what I had said. She was just opening an envelope with the results of lab tests after a total checkup. What I said to her matched the lab report precisely, down to indicating that she was dangerously low in potassium. This was the event, more than even the healing, that made her accept Balasheem. She called him her personal angel and embraced him into her belief system.

My next trip to teach in San Diego was that summer. I was driving south on Highway 5, my daughters Tanya and Dondi were sleeping in the back seat, and it was raining heavily. We had just passed through Sacramento when suddenly I saw the figure of Balasheem outside the windshield. He told me to call Betty. "Tell her, that which just happened is not her fault."

In the most painful corners of our experience something alive always wants to come forth, as the poet Rilke suggests: "Perhaps all the dragons in our lives are princesses who are only waiting to see us act just once, with beauty and courage. Perhaps everything that frightens us is, in its deeper essence, something helpless that needs our love." So whatever pain or problem we have, if it helps us find a quality of presence—where we can open to it, see it, feel it, include it, and find the truth concealed in it—that is our healing.

—John Welwood

I anxiously drove to a phone and called. A man answered, and I asked to speak with Betty. He said, "I'm sorry, you can't speak with her right now." I said, "Please, I must speak with her." He said, "It's impossible! Please call back later." "No, I must speak with her now. Please tell Betty this is Donna, and I have spoken to Balasheem."

When he told her it was me, she came to the phone. I began, "Betty, don't say anything," and I told her how Balasheem had come in front of the windshield and told me to tell her "That which has just happened is not your fault." She let out a scream and began to sob. Someone was trying to take the phone away from her, and Betty was saying, "No, no!" Then a peace seemed to come over her. She asked if he had said anything more. I said, "Not yet, but I'm on my way to San Diego. Betty, what is it?"

"My son just killed himself."

I went straight to Betty's house when I arrived in San Diego. She was sleeping. Her husband told me she was having heart irregularities before my call, but she was calmer now. He spoke of their shock and guilt. Betty's love for this son was both boundless and agonizingly complicated, but the husband's grief was made worse because he and the son had been estranged. Betty had been placed in the middle, forcing herself to assume a "tough love" attitude that went against her maternal instincts.

I heard Betty stir and went in to see her. The room was filled with so much love and tenderness that, before I saw him, I knew Balasheem was present. Emanating from him was a phenomenal compassion and reverence for the gravity of the situation. I felt privy to something extraordinarily intimate. I said, "Betty, he's here."

Remarkable information began to come forth. The son's body was in such bad shape from years of drug abuse that he would have, in any event, died within a couple of years of liver disease. He had the kind of body chemistry that simply could not afford to trifle with drugs. But by stepping out of his life at this time, he felt he was preventing harm from coming to those he loved as he recognized that he could not stop himself from doing horrendous things to get drugs. He chose suicide as the less terrible alternative. This blew me away. I do not condone suicide. It goes so strongly against my instincts that I had a hard time reconciling myself to Balasheem's words.

For the next three days, I saw Betty each day, and Balasheem appeared each time. He explained that for the entire year before the suicide, it appeared unstoppable. *That* was the reason Balasheem had first "tapped Donna on the shoulder" to make his presence known to Betty. Healing Betty's body was the vehicle to make contact and gain her trust as a larger story was unfolding. It became clear to Balasheem that Betty's heart would not survive her son's suicide. So Balasheem began to create conditions that would minimize the wider damage of the inevitable suicide.

During the third session with Betty, she gasped, "I see him! I SEE YOU!!!" She began to speak with and hear Balasheem, and I was no longer the intermediary. But it was her son's voice that she really wanted to hear. Her heart was so burdened from missing him that she could not stop the pain. Every day for six months she went to his grave, leaving him fresh flowers. One day, after she had spoken to him, cried for him, and put the flowers down, she turned to leave and heard his voice as distinctly as if he were standing behind her. He said, "Oh, Mom, take the flowers home and enjoy them." The terrible agony of her grief was lifted. . . .

Poignant encounters with invisible spirits, previous lifetimes, and voices of the deceased who provide verifiable information tend to open one's metaphysical perspective. I am certain that the soul passes through other realms that we can only glimpse. These glimpses, however, seem to offer a natural if unconventional source of information. Such information has again and again provided me with a key for unlocking a healing process, occasionally in individuals who have been abandoned as beyond hope by Western medicine, its true marvels notwithstanding.

So how do I make sense of bizarre encounters such as those with the likes of Balasheem? There is no question in my mind that these exceptional realms are just as "real," just as valid, as anything in the ordinary physical world, and that the principles governing them are just as lawful. Tuning into these more elusive zones has provided me with a deeper understanding about healing by placing illness into the larger context of the soul's journey, and it has consistently made my own life a more magical voyage.

I, in fact, love being tuned into that realm. From it I feel in touch with deeper truths and truer perceptions. I see beauty and perfection. I'm always ready for the unexpected, and it may appear in the most interesting and gratifying ways. At such moments I enter a state of deep appreciation of life and its many wonders. I become more accessible to a Balasheem and more open to subtle knowledge about the nature of things. To simply imagine this mystical zone is a knock on its door. To actively pursue it is a turn of the key. If you frequent this world—pursuing and entering it through meditation, ritual, sacred plants, healing work, or spontaneous grace—you know that my attempt here to capture it with words is inadequate. If you do not, knock at its door from time to time as you go through your week, and be receptive to the advent of mystery.

HELPING PATIENTS
DECIDE TO DIE

M. Scott Peck

MALCOLM MORRISON WAS NOT A HYPOTHETICAL CASE.
I was asked to consult on the case in the early 1980s, toward the conclusion of my psychiatric practice. The formal request came from the oncologist at the hospital where Malcolm was an inpatient, but I was informed it was actually initiated by Malcolm's wife, Betty.

Malcolm had been diagnosed as having inoperable cancer of the lung two years previously when he was sixty-five. At the time I was asked to see him, he was undergoing his third course of radiation therapy, and the radiologist had reported that his massive tumor had possibly begun to shrink slightly once again in response. Only Malcolm had almost stopped eating. The oncologist explained to Betty that, despite the equivocally positive radiology report, Malcolm would die if he couldn't become better nourished. She asked if a psychiatrist could be called in to discover why he wasn't eating.

There is a medical term for the wasting of the body that so often accompanies cancer and a few other conditions: cachexia. Literally it means "bad disease." It is as if the cancer has run wild and is consuming all the patient's nutrition and sapping the healthy tissues as well. Cachexia may range from mild to severe. When mild, the patient may look

Right: Burning Man 2001, Photography by Tony Pletts. This bier at the Burning Man Festival invited festival goers to examine their own mortality.

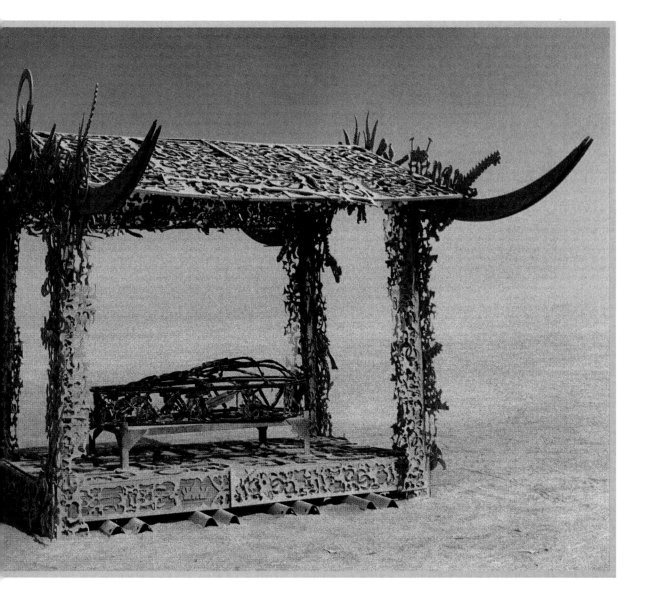

perfectly well nourished, but there is a certain slight sunkenness to the cheeks and a subtle sense of shadow descending upon the body. When severe, the patient has wasted away to little more than a skeleton. I began my consultation simply by looking at Malcolm lying in bed from the distance of his hospital room doorway. I'd never seen a human being more cachectic. I'd also never known a cancer patient so cachectic to survive.

Since she had been the one to request my services, I next went to talk to Betty in the waiting room, aware that there were at least three possible purely physical reasons why Malcolm wasn't eating that had nothing to do with psychiatry. Betty was a robust, deeply caring woman in her sixties. I took an instant liking to her. Interspersed between her comments on the details of the case, she said, "It's been a long battle, but we'll win it yet. I know it looks bad right now, but Malcolm's a fighter. Together we're going to beat this thing. Neither of us is a quitter." The military analogies went on and on.

Finally I said with trepidation, "Betty, it's clear to me that your fighting spirit, in conjunction with Malcolm's, is what has kept him alive for so long. You've done a wonderful and heroic job. But I'm not sure that now is the time for fighting. I wonder if the most loving thing you could do for Malcolm at this point wouldn't be to give him your permission to die, if that's what he wants. Is that something you'd be willing to consider?"

Clearly this was a shock to her, but yes, Betty said, it was something she would think about. It was now Monday noon; I made an appointment to meet her at the hospital again early Wednesday morning.

Next I went to talk with Malcolm. It was painful to look into eyes so sunken, and difficult to understand a voice so weak. But he was quite lucid. He didn't really know why he wasn't eating, he explained. He didn't actually feel an obstruction; he simply had no appetite. No, it was worse than that. That he could overcome. But whenever he forced himself to take a mouthful of food he felt absolute repugnance at the thought of taking a second.

The final step in the healing process is to open our heart to the vicissitudes we are facing in our lives. A friend who was dying of cancer tried every possible treatment she could find. Nothing worked. Finally she realized that the real healing was not in curing the cancer but in coming to terms with it. That was actually a much greater kind of healing.

—John Welwood

"You must be tired," I said.

He acknowledged he was.

"Would you like to die?" I asked. "Do you feel like giving up?"

A spasm of fear, almost panic, crossed Malcolm's face. "No," he exclaimed, "I don't want to die. I'll eat. I'll make myself eat. I'm not a quitter."

"You sound as if it's bad to quit," I commented.

Those sunken eyes looked up at me with such surprise it was almost like a glimmer of light. "Isn't it?" he asked.

"Isn't it bad to quit?" I repeated.

"Yes. Isn't it?"

"Sometimes yes, sometimes no," I answered him. "When I was fifteen I quit a school where I'd been very unhappy for over two years. At the time I felt guilty for not toughing it out, but now when I look back on it I think it was the best decision I ever made in my life. I'm also here seeing you today as a country psychiatrist only because ten years ago I quit a government job in Washington. Although I was exhausted, I again felt guilty—this time for letting the government down. But the government could go on without me, and I'm glad I did it, and I'm glad I'm here with you now.

"I'm not saying that quitting is good, Malcolm," I continued. "It might just be the wrong thing to do. And I can't tell you what to do in your case. It's a terribly difficult decision, and it's entirely yours to make. All I can tell you is that it's not necessarily bad to quit."

With that I left.

When I returned to see her on Wednesday morning, Betty said, "Malcolm and I have done a lot of praying and crying together these past thirty-six hours. We've decided to go home today. In fact, they're preparing Malcolm now." I told her I thought it was a courageous decision.

Early Friday evening Betty called to tell me Malcolm had died peacefully at home that morning. I wrote her a note of condolence. Two weeks later I received a note back from her thanking me for my service. I felt as proud of that brief service as any other in my career as a psychiatrist and physician.

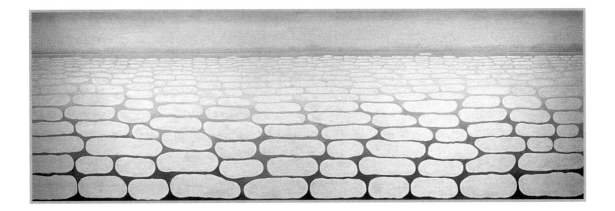

W I S T E R I A

Leslie Nyman

A SHUDDER OF RESISTANCE SHIVERED THROUGH ME AS I RAN TOWARD THE OLD BRICK HOSPITAL. NOVEMBER'S ICY RAIN had stripped the last of the wisteria from the vines covering the stone-gray building. In spring, when I began my nursing career, the smell of these purple flowers filled the air; now the chill dampness of late autumn drained scent and color into memory.

Cold winds pushed me into the lighted entry hall where my coworkers, Alma and Rosy, were already shaking off the chill.

"Ah, rain. No me le gusto, sí? I don't like esta noche."

Alma chattered "Spanglish," her concession to a common language, and Rosy ignored me with her usual benign indulgence. Even though we shared jokes, coffee and donuts, and complaints about hospital policies, Rosy closed herself off to me.

Above: Georgia O'Keeffe, *Sky Above Clouds IV.* Death is sometimes described as dissolution into the wide blue sky. **Right:** Georgia O'Keeffe, *Blue and Green Music.* In this painting the artist played with the translation of the intangibility of music into color and form. The story also deals with an intangible sense—smell and its evocative nature.

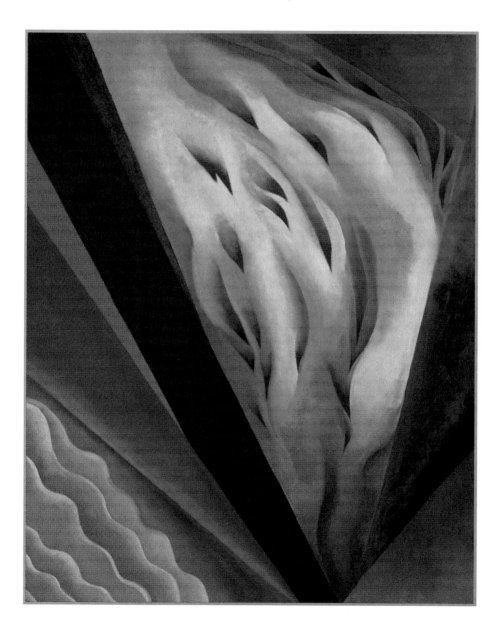

"Bad storm tonight." I fumbled for a pen and paper while Louise, the evening-shift nurse, paced around the small enclosure of desk, chart rack, and medicine cabinet.

"The first storms of the season are always the worst. November sets a chill in my bones that doesn't leave until May." She pulled on her rubber overshoes. "Come on, let's get report started so I can go home to a hot tub."

Before sitting down, I turned on the hall light and the second set of office lights. "It feels creepy in here tonight."

"This place can spook you until you get used to it," she laughed. "Wait until you've been around fourteen years, like me. Nothing about this place bothers me anymore."

I aspired to Louise's cool professionalism. She possessed the emotional distance that I believed distinguished the most competent nurses. She reported on the patients' conditions like a child reciting a poem. The rhythm pulled the matter-of-fact words along.

"Mr. Edwards' ulcer is worse today. Try to change his position every two hours tonight. Miss Wallace is going to the general hospital in the A.M. for a biopsy." She looked up as if to say *at last* but merely shook her head and continued her report. "Mary Cromer refused to eat again today. Maybe it's time for a feeding tube. . . or a psych consult. I left her doctor a note. John Kline . . . ," she broke the rhythm with a deep sigh. "John needed morphine twice on my time, twice on the day shift. He seems to be getting worse. The morphine barely holds him for four hours." She lit a cigarette. "Can you believe it, Janie? This is still a PRN order." Exhaling a cloud of smoke, she leaned toward me confidentially. "You know, I think his doctor is afraid John will get addicted if we give it around the clock. The poor guy probably doesn't have another month to go. I wish we could keep him comfortable." Crushing out the half-smoked cigarette, she stood abruptly. "Everyone else on the floor is stable. Come on, let's make rounds so I can get out of here."

I followed Louise in and out of the dim rooms as she made a final check at each bedside. I made notes of the bags, bottles, and tubes that were to occupy my hours. The rooms were populated with sleeping, groaning, babbling patients.

"Hey you, get me up! I've got to get . . . ouch, ouch."

"Now, now Betty, wherever do you have to get to at this hour?"

Louise teased the shrunken, wrinkled lady in bed.

"Get away, girl," the old woman spit. "My leg hurts, my leg." Louise and I freed Betty from the tangle of sheets. We moved pillows behind her back and between her knees, arranging her in a more comfortable position.

"There, isn't that better now, dear?" Louise cooed. As we left the room Louise told me, "Betty's getting crazier by the day. She's totally out of it. She talks all day to her dead husband, doesn't even recognize her son when he visits". I guess she keeps the day shift entertained." She shrugged. "Anyway, I hope you have a quiet night. I'm free at last."

Gray light, like evening fog, settled in the hospital corridors. Only the absence of darkness lightened the hallways. The rowdy storm outside rattled the window but did not disturb the palpable rhythm of the midnight quiet. It felt as though everyone was inhaling at the same time and slowly exhaling together.

At one A.M. rounds everyone was stable. Mr. Edwards had been turned on his side. Alma and Rosy cleaned up soiled patients, changed linens, added a needed blanket, and restrained a restless sleeper. I liked the pace of the night shift as it moved through its hours with the steady ticking of a clock. My only concern was that someone would die. No one had ever died on my shift. I felt a combination of shame and eagerness as I stood over a faltering patient, hoping he or she would live until eight A.M. Death scared me. I had no experience with it and thought of it as something ugly, painful, and vaguely contagious.

"Help me, help me please," a small voice cried.

"There go Betty otra vez. I change her sheets, but it no calm her. She unhappy vieja." Alma snapped her gum.

I did not know what more I could offer. She had already been given her tranquilizer for the night. "Maybe I'll sit with her awhile," I said to Rosy. She nodded.

"Oh dear, I'm so afraid." Betty's voice shook.

"It's OK, you're safe," I reassured her, stroking her large gnarled

From the middle of life onward, only he remains vitally alive who is ready to die with life.

—Carl Gustav Jung

hands. Long ago they must have been useful and perhaps lovely, but now the nails were yellowed and splintered. I wondered about the crooked tip of her index finger. It looked as if it had been broken and never set right.

"They've all left me. I'm all alone," she cried. "Oh Charles. He never would let them do this to me. He never let me be alone so." The depth of her sigh caused a wheeze.

"What was Charles like?" I asked, knowing that by talking about him she might find solace.

"He was a good man. You know, a *real* man." Her thin voice pretended strength. "So handsome. All the other girls were jealous." Her eyes twinkled. "Yes, everyone looked up to him."

Before leaving the room I stroked her soft white hair. She had fallen back to what I hoped was a pleasant dream.

Wind and rain tapped a lullaby on the window panes. Three A.M. was always a difficult hour for me to keep my eyes open. I walk through the rooms, stopping at each bedside, wondering what the patients' lives had been before illness and age had wasted them. I made sure the bedrails were up and that everyone was breathing.

John Kline was awake.

"The pain's comin' in waves." A shadow of playfulness lingered about his mouth. "I'm waitin' ta see what crests with the next wave."

He stopped talking, eyes closed and lips taut. My fingertips resting on his wrist felt his pulse increase with the pain.

"No ship in sight. Send for the Marines. Suppose I could have my medicine now?"

It had been the required four hours since his last shot. "The Marines have landed," I whispered as I administered the morphine. Tomorrow the nurses could do battle with the doctor for more ammunition against John's pain.

A bedrail rattled in the next room. I found Betty half turned around in bed, mumbling to herself.

"Get me out of here! I want to see my Charles." A trace of anger flickered. "He'd get me out of here!" her gray eyes misted. "I don't know what happened." She slid back into confusion. "Joey used to be a good boy, but then Charles died and, I don't know . . ." Her uncomprehending eyes looked to me. "Dear, do I know you? What's your name?"

"Janie. My name is Janie and I'm your nurse."

"My nurse?" She was indignant in an instant. "I don't need a nurse. I've always been the healthiest of all my sisters—Sadie, she's the sick one. What do I need a nurse for?"

"Betty, it's hard for you to walk, and your family wants you to be safe and cared for."

"I don't need to be taken care of," she snapped. "Joey's always helped me. It's only right. I looked after my mother 'til the day she died." Betty turned her face away from me. "It's not right, it's just not right." She lifted her big hands to reveal their emptiness. "But I can tell you one thing." Her steely eyes turned to me. "If Charles were here, things would be different. He'd tell you and your people to go to hell."

Pride slipped into weariness. Paper-thin eyelids closed. Her wheezing filled the room.

"Please, don't go yet." She placed her knobby hand over mine. "Oh mama," her tiny voice cracked.

The building shivered in the cold wind. I heard Rosy exclaim, "Lord, what a night!" from down the hall. Icy rain slamming into the sill startled Betty.

"Quick, answer the door. I wonder who that could be?"

"It's only the weather, that's all. A storm," I whispered.

"A storm? I didn't know. I must watch for Charles. My glasses. I can't see. Where are my glasses?"

I placed very smudged bifocals on her shrunken face. In the dim hospital light she looked like an owl—eyes wide open looking into the night.

"Now dear, help me to the window. I've got to get to the window. Charles will be home soon." She pulled up her knees to swing herself out of bed. Her ankle fell between the bars of the siderail.

I untied the knot she had made with her legs, the siderail, and the linens, and helped her to sit on the edge of the bed, the flat of my hand supporting her bent back. She felt like nothing more than a bundle of twigs.

"Let's sit here a moment and rest."

"I've rested enough," she growled, her heavy hand pressed into my knee for leverage as she stood. It was a slow shuffle to the window. I tried to surround her thin body with my arms, my feet close to her leaden steps as she dragged across the linoleum floor, filling the room with her whistle and wheeze. Fixing her magnified gray eyes on a point on the window, she drew nearer as if guided by an invisible pulley. Goosebumps crawled over my skin and my palms were sweating, but I held her up as we proceeded. I craned my neck back toward the door, hoping that Rosy or Alma would appear. I never should have let this happen, but Betty's insistence was stronger than my fear.

Her long crooked fingers clung to the windowsill like a bird to a branch. I supported her waist while she leaned forward to peer out.

"I can see him coming up the road." Her frail body tensed with excitement.

I looked out the window. It was a dark night; the branches blowing against the pane were barely visible.

Betty stared hard into the night. "Oh, he works so hard, that old guy," she whispered. Her voice lightened into a song, almost a laugh. "Quick, Joey, can you smell the wisteria? It's so sweet."

Then she sank, quickly, painlessly into my arms. I nearly dropped her I was so surprised. In the breath of the second that precedes a thought, I understood—death had relieved her. The complete stillness when her wheezing ceased scared me. I struggled to carry her now-heavy body to the bed.

Deafened by the pounding of my own heart, I ran to find Alma and Rosy.

"I shouldn't have let her out of bed! I knew it!" Tears showed my confusion. "This never happened to me before." I searched their faces for a suggestion of what to do.

"Janie, calm yourself." Alma wrapped her long arm around my shoulders. "She was una vieja." She shrugged. "She died, rest her soul in heaven. We will finish the colecciones and IV for you while you take care of business." When she kissed my cheek I smelled her flowery perfume that had not faded during the night.

"You know," I said to Rosy, whose eyes revealed compassion, "she said she saw her husband. That was all she seemed to want really. I'm sort of glad, if she saw him like that, you know, at the end."

Rosy's smile offered me a moment of comfort.

"I don't know, I don't know." I paced in a tight circle. "Am I responsible?"

"No, Janie, you didn't do nothing. The old lady died because it was God's will, not yours. That mean old lady is in everlasting peace right now. She's not a joke for nobody."

Rosy's words helped to calm me into reason. The necessary phone calls were made, the paperwork completed.

As dawn ignited the dark sky, the sounds of early risers could be heard. Old machines cranking their engines, doubtful people looking to see if they were still alive, and groaning as they realized they had awakened into their nightmare. I opened the window in Betty's room. The storm was ending. Wet earth perfumed the cold air. Winter was coming, but for a moment I could almost smell the wisteria.

Right: Sarah Pletts, *Warped Fruit III.*

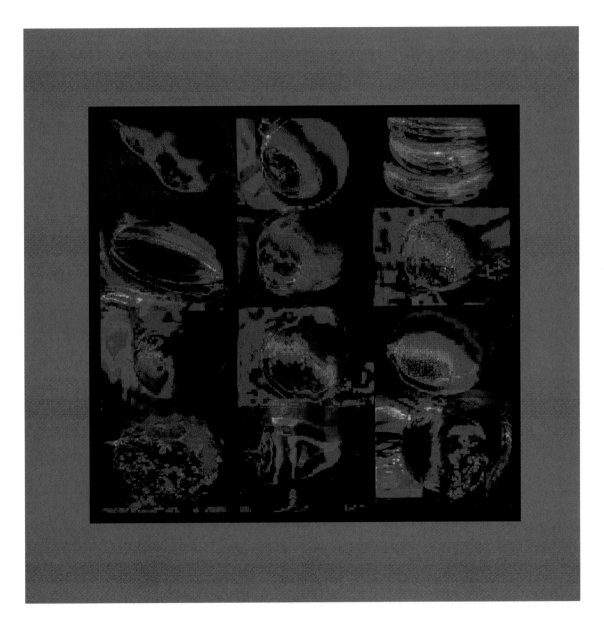

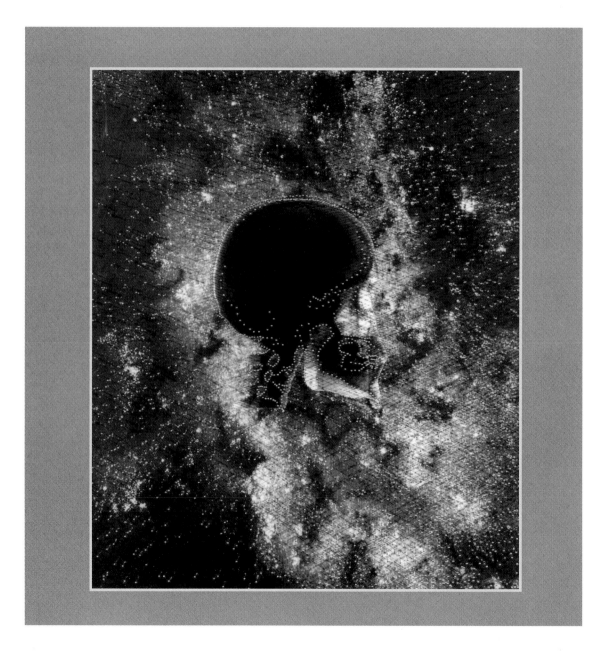

THE FINAL LESSON

Rachel Naomi Remem

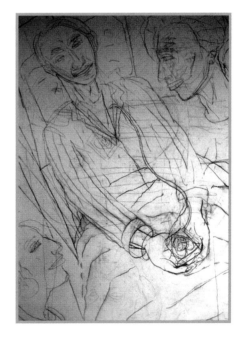

S OMETIMES THE PARTICULARS OF THE WAY IN WHICH SOMEONE dies, the time, place, even the circumstances, may cause those left behind to wonder whether the event marks the healing of hidden patterns and personal issues, and answers for that person certain lifelong questions. Death has been referred to as the great teacher. It may be the great healer as well. *Educare*, the root word of 'education,' means to lead forth the innate wholeness in a person. So, in the deepest sense, that which truly educates us also heals us.

The theory of karma suggests that life itself is in its essential nature both educational and healing, that the innate wholeness underlying the personality of each of us is being evoked, clarified, and strengthened through the challenges and

Left: Lucas Samaras, *Skull & Milky Way*. This artwork suggests both our mortality and meeting with something greater than ourselves as we return to the stardust from which we came.
Right: Sarah Pletts, *Intensive Care*.

experiences of our lifetime. All life paths may be a movement toward the soul. In which case our death may be the final and most integrating of our life's experiences.

When I met Thomas, he was over seventy, a family-practice physician who had been in solo practice for almost fifty years. Whole families, from grandparents to grandchildren, looked to him for help in their troubles, counted on his counsel, and called him their friend. He looked the part too, gray-haired, kindly, his body as spare and gnarled as an old oak.

At the time that we met, he had end-stage lung cancer. He could no longer get around without the constant flow of oxygen through a nasal catheter, and the previous month he had closed his medical practice. Until the last year he had never missed a day. An astute diagnostician, he had come because he knew he was dying. He proposed that we open a series of conversations about his life. He had done some reflection in recent years but felt that sharing the process at this point might be helpful in readying himself for death.

Thomas felt death to be an unqualified ending to life. Raised a Catholic, he had left the church early and embraced science as a way to bring order to the chaos of life. It had not failed him. Yet life had intrinsic value for him and he wished to examine and understand his own life and what it had meant.

It surprised me that a man this altruistic, compassionate, and reverent toward the life in others, this awed by the beauty of anatomy and physiology, held no religious or spiritual beliefs. Curious, I asked him about the circumstances under which he had decided to leave the church. Open and frank about other details of his long life, he was reticent in the extreme about this. He had left at sixteen over a specific happening. I never found out what it was.

Thomas had been a loner all his life. Never married, he had led a personal life that was solitary almost to the point of asceticism. Yet he was a

I have heard of many cases of people who were diagnosed as terminally ill and given only a few months to live. When they went into solitude, followed a spiritual practice, and truly faced themselves and the fact of death, they were healed. What is this telling us? That when we accept death, transform our attitude toward life, and discover the fundamental connection between life and death, a dramatic possibility for healing can occur. . . .

Illnesses like cancer can be a warning, to remind us that we have been neglecting deep aspects of our being, such as our spiritual needs. If we take this warning seriously and change fundamentally the direction of our lives, there is a very real hope for healing not only our bodies, but our whole being.

—Sogyal Rimpoche

connoisseur of beauty in all its forms, a patron of the arts, poetry, theater, music, ballet, and literature. His library held over a thousand books. Thomas's major commitment was to his medicine, his families and their needs, hopes, and dreams. His devotion to them was absolute.

Very early on in our discussions, I asked him how he saw his relationship to his patients. Looking at a small figurine of a shepherd with his flock that another patient had given me, he smiled. "Like that." We spent the next few weeks examining the nature of his work and what it had meant to him. The shepherd was a steward of the life in the flock, he protected them from danger, helped them to find nurture and fulfill themselves. He delivered their young. He found the strays and brought them back to the others.

Thomas told me many stories of his shepherding and the life of his flock. We examined these stories together, sharing our thoughts and perspectives. In the telling and the reflection, he seemed to be unfolding a much deeper sense of what his life had meant to others and what he had stood for. In these discussions, he often used an odd Victorian word: they "sheltered" with him. He was their safety, their support, their friend. He was there for them, constant, vigilant, and trustworthy. We discussed the yang or masculine principle of action and protection and the yin or feminine principle of acceptance and nurture and how these came together in the person of a shepherd. The symbol emerged as a symbol of wholeness.

All the while, he was becoming more and more ill, his breathing more labored. Eventually I raised the issue of his personal isolation. Who did he shelter with, who was the shepherd's shepherd? "No one," he said, the words holding more pain than he had expressed before. It became clear that he did not believe that there was a place of sheltering for himself. Shepherd though he was professionally, personally he had become separated from the flock, a nonparticipant, a lost person. He seemed unwilling to go much further with this.

Puzzled, I asked him to make up a story about a lost lamb, and haltingly he described a lamb that had been lost for so long that he could not even remember there was a flock. He had learned to survive by himself, to eat what was available, to hide from predators. "Does this lamb know that his shepherd is looking for him?" I asked. "No," he said, "the lamb had done something very bad and the shepherd had forgotten him."

"As a shepherd yourself, would you look for a lost lamb who had done something bad?" He seemed puzzled. I reminded him of the young patient from the projects he had told me about, the one he had taken on as a guardian from the juvenile courts, the girl who eventually went on to college. I asked him why he had gone after her and brought her home. "Why, she was one of mine," he said unhesitatingly. "Yes," I said. There was a small silence. Then he abruptly changed the subject, but I saw he was deeply affected by the thought that the bond between the shepherd and his sheep might lie beyond judgment and was deeper than he had previously thought.

We talked of many other things over the next months and gradually the image of the shepherd retreated to the back of my mind. We spoke of childhood and manhood and lost love, and the richness of seventy years of living became apparent to us both. It had been a good life.

Thomas was hospitalized once and his health continued to worsen. His oncologist had exhausted all treatment for his cancer and began to increase medications to ease his respiratory distress. Gradually he became too ill to come to the office and in the fall I began to see him at his home. Hospice was called and by the beginning of December he had become so short of breath that he could no longer speak. I sat with him and held his hand. Sometimes I would read him poetry or sing to him a little.

Somehow he kept hanging on. The hospice workers were surprised by his endurance. One of his nurses told me that she thought he was waiting for something. I thought perhaps she was right but I had no idea of what it could be. His brother had come from the East Coast to say good-bye and many of his patients had already visited and left cards and other expressions of their love.

On Christmas Eve I received a call from his nurse. Thomas had been in a coma all day and now he was having difficulty with his secretions. Would I come? As soon as I saw Thomas, I realized that he was dying. His breathing, always labored, had become shallow and intermittent. The nurse with him was young and seemed a little uncertain and so I invited her to stay as I talked to him. He did not respond in any way. We changed his sheets and made him more comfortable. Then we sat down together to wait. Gradually the space between his breaths lengthened and after a while his breathing stopped.

The young nurse seemed relieved. She called Thomas's brother, who had asked to be notified and who said that he would fly out the next day. He asked that she call the funeral director Thomas had chosen and she called him, too. She called his oncologist to sign the death certificate. There seemed nothing more to do. I stood for a time at the foot of Thomas's bed, thinking about him and wishing him well. Then I left.

It was dark and had grown quite cold. Holding my keys in my pocket, I huddled into my coat and walked a little faster. I had almost reached my car when church bells throughout the city began ringing. For a moment I stopped, confused. Could they be ringing for Thomas? And then I remembered. It was midnight. The Shepherd had come.

Right: Georgia O'Keeffe, *Black Rock with Blue Sky and White Clouds.*

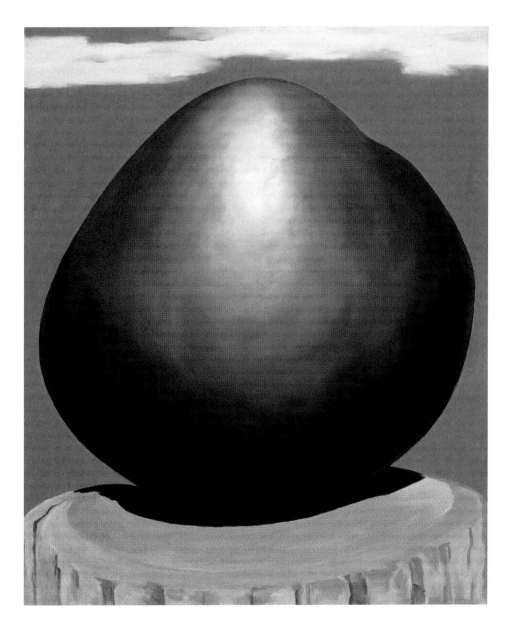

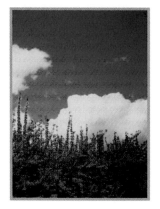

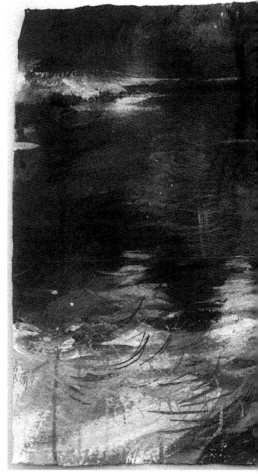

STILL HERE

Ram Dass

ONE EVENING IN FEBRUARY 1997, I WAS IN BED AT HOME IN Marin County, contemplating how to end my book. I'd been working on the manuscript for eighteen months, weaving together material from personal experience and from talks I'd given around the country on conscious aging, but somehow the book's conclusion had eluded me. Lying there in the dark, I wondered why what I'd written seemed so incomplete, not quite rounded,

Above: Photograph by Andrew Lane.   **Right:** Nick Andrew, *Chirallo.* The serenity of the painting echoes the calmness that can come with the attitude of acceptance in the text.

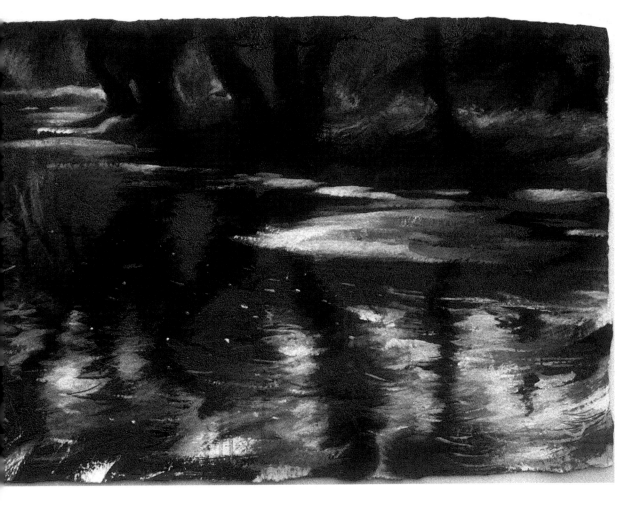

grounded, or whole. I tried to imagine what life would be like if I were *very* old—not an active person of sixty-five, traveling the world incessantly as a teacher and speaker, caught up in my public role—but as someone of ninety, say, with failing sight and failing limbs. I fantasized how that old man would think, how he'd move and speak and hear, what desires he might have as he slowly surveyed the world. I was trying to *feel* my way into oldness. I was thoroughly enjoying this fantasy when the phone rang. In the process of my fantasy, I'd noticed that my leg seemed to have fallen asleep. As I got up to answer the phone, my leg gave way under me and I fell to the floor. In my mind, the fall was still part of my "old man fantasy." I didn't realize that my leg was no longer working because I'd had a stroke.

I reached for my phone, on the table near my bed.

"R. D.? Are you there?"

I heard the voice of an old friend in Santa Fe. When I didn't respond coherently, he asked, "Are you sick?" I suppose I still didn't answer, so he said, "If you can't speak, tap on the phone. Tap once for yes and twice for no." When he asked whether I wanted help, I tapped "no" over and over again.

Nonetheless, he contacted my secretaries, who live close by, and the next thing I knew they rushed into the house and found me on the floor. There I was flat on my back, still caught in my "dream" of the very old man, who had now fallen down because his leg wouldn't work. My assistants seemed very frightened; they called 911. My next recollection is of a group of young firemen, straight out of central casting, staring into the old man's face while I observed the whole thing as if from a doorway to the side. I'm told I was immediately rushed to a hospital nearby, but all I remember is being rolled down the hospital corridors, looking up at the ceiling pipes and the concerned faces of nurses and friends. I was fascinated by what was happening.

Only afterward did I learn that I had a stroke and realize how close to death I had actually been. The doctors told my friends I had a massive cerebral hemorrhage, and only a ten percent chance of survival. I noticed the looks of deep concern on the faces of the doctors and my friends, but the thought of dying was nowhere in my mind, so I was perplexed by their grave expressions.

Three hospitals and hundreds of hours of rehabilitation later, I gradually eased into my new post-stroke life as someone in a wheelchair, partially paralyzed, requiring round-the-clock care and a degree of personal attention that made me uncomfortable. All my life I had been a "helper"; I had even collaborated on a book called *How Can I Help?* I now found myself forced to accept the help of others, and to admit that my body needed attention. Because I'd spent my adult life concentrating on the realms of the spirit, I'd always been able to rationalize the distance I maintained from my body by saying that my detachment was a spiritual witnessing of the physical form. But that had been only partly true. The truth is that I distanced myself from my body. I saw my body as merely a vehicle for the soul. I ignored it as much as possible and tried to spiritualize it away.

From a physical perspective, the lack of love I'd shown toward my body contributed to my stroke. I was negligent about taking my blood pressure medicine and, a month before the stroke, ignored an unusual one-side hearing loss while scuba diving in the Caribbean. Before the stroke, although I was in my 60's, I saw myself as young and powerful, with my MG, golf clubs, surfing, and speaking gigs. Illness had shattered my self-image, and opened the door to a new chapter in my life.

After any major physical "insult," as they call it, it's all too easy to see yourself as a collection of symptoms rather than as a total human being, including your spirit—and thus to become your illness. Fear is powerful and contagious, and at first I allowed myself to catch it, worried that if I didn't do what the doctors ordered, I'd be sorry. But now I'm learning to take my healing into my own hands. Healing is not the same as curing, after all; healing does not mean going back to the way things were before, but rather allowing *what is now* to move us closer to God.

For example, since my speech was severely impaired by this stroke, I considered not speaking publicly anymore, since the words came so slowly, but people insisted that my halting new voice enabled them to concentrate on the silence between the words. Now that I speak more slowly, people tend to finish my sentences for me, and thus to answer questions for themselves. Though I once used silence as a teaching method, it now arises without my control and allows for a sense of emptiness, an emptiness that listeners can use as a doorway to their inner quiet.

My guru once said to a visitor complaining about her suffering, "I

The more I work with the body, keeping my assumptions in a temporary state of reservation, the more I appreciate and sympathize with a given disease. The body no longer appears as a sick or irrational demon, but as a process with its own inner logic and wisdom.

—Thomas Arnold Mitchell

love suffering. It brings me so close to God." In this same way, I've learned that the incidents associated with aging—including this stroke—can be used for our spiritual healing, provided we learn to see through new eyes.

Although my outward life has been radically altered, I don't see myself as a stroke victim. I see myself as a Soul who's watching "him" experience the aftermath of this cerebral hemorrhage. Having accepted my predicament, I'm much happier than I was before. This troubles some of the people around me. They have told me that I should fight to walk again, but I don't know if I wanted to walk. I'm sitting—that's where I am. I'm peaceful like this and I am grateful to the people who care for me. Why is this wrong? Though I can now stand and move around with a walker, I've grown to love my wheelchair (I call it my swan boat) and being wheeled about by people who care. They carry Chinese emperors and Indian *maharajas* on palanquins; in other cultures, it's a symbol of honor and power to be carried and wheeled. I don't believe it's all-important to be what our culture calls "optimal."

Before the stroke I wrote a great deal about the terrible things that can happen in aging, and how to cope with them. Now I'm happy to say that having gone through what some would view as the worst, it's not so bad after all.

Getting old isn't easy for a lot of us. Neither is living, neither is dying. We struggle against the inevitable and we all suffer because of it. We have to find another way to look at the whole process of being born, growing old, changing, and dying, some kind of perspective that might allow us to deal with what we perceive as big obstacles without having to be dragged through the drama. It really helps to understand that we have something—that we *are* something—which is unchangeable, beautiful, completely aware, and continues no matter what. Knowing this doesn't solve everything—this is what I encountered and told about in *Be Here Now*, and I've still had my share of suffering. But the perspective of the soul can help a lot with the little things, and it is my hope that you'll be able to from this take book some joy in being "still here."

Recently, a friend said to me, "You're more human since the stroke than you were before." This touched me profoundly. What a gift the stroke has given me, to finally learn that I don't have to renounce my humanity in order to he spiritual—that I can be both witness and participant, both eternal spirit and aging body. The book's ending, which had eluded me, is now finally clear. The stroke has given me a new perspective to share about aging, a perspective that says, "Don't be a wise elder, be an incarnation of wisdom." That changes the whole nature of the game. That's not just a new role, it's a new state of being. It's the real thing. At nearly seventy, surrounded by people who care for and love me, I'm still learning to be here now.

Right: Julian Onderdonk, *A Cloudy Day, Bluebonnets near San Antonio, Texas.*

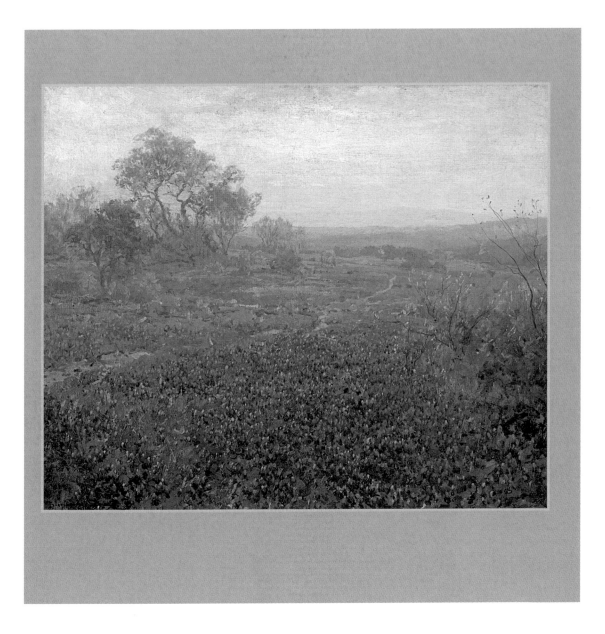

ACKNOWLEDGMENTS

First and foremost, we would like to thank Jeremy Tarcher for his vision in creating this anthology series, and for his dedication and unwavering support in guiding the book towards completion. Our greatest appreciation is also extended to Robert Bly, Jean Houston, Robert A. Johnson, and Andrew Weil for their essential contributions to this series. To John Beebe, editor of the *San Francisco Institute Library Journal,* Alan B. Chinen, Connie Zweig, and the many members of the Jungian, transpersonal, and holistic medicine communities for their insights and suggestions concerning the selection of materials for these books—our deepest thanks. The talents of several people came together to make this unique collection of stories and art into the beautiful volume you hold in your hands. Mark Robert Waldman, whose skills as an author and editor shine in the choices he made for the book, carefully selected the texts. Julie Foakes, whose talents as an art researcher can never be praised enough, chose all the images. Marion Kocot brought order and harmony to the words with her talented editing skills. Sara Carder at Tarcher Putnam provided constant encouragement and handholding throughout the process. Joel Fontinos, the publisher at Tarcher Putnam, guided us with enthusiasm and praise. And Kristen Garneau brought text and images together in the elegant layout of the pages. To you all A HUGE THANK YOU!

—Philip and Manuela Dunn of The Book Laboratory Inc.

ABOUT THE EDITOR

Mark Robert Waldman is a therapist and the author and editor of numerous books, including *The Spirit of Writing, Love Games, Dreamscaping* and *The Art of Staying Together*. He was founding editor of *Transpersonal Review*, covering the fields of transpersonal and Jungian psychology, religious studies, and mind/body medicine.

ABOUT THE BOOK CREATORS

Philip Dunn and Manuela Dunn Mascetti have created many best-selling volumes, including *The Illustrated Rumi*, Huston Smith's *Illustrated World's Religions*, Stephen Hawking's *The Illustrated A Brief History of Time* and *The Universe in a Nutshell*, and Thomas Moore's *The Illustrated Care of the Soul*. They are the authors of *The Illustrated Rumi, The Buddha Box*, and many other books.

ABOUT THE INTRODUCTORY AUTHOR

Andrew Weil, M. D. , is a clinical professor of internal medicine as well as the founder and the director of the Program of Integrative Medicine at the University of Arizona's Health Sciences Center in Tucson. A graduate of Harvard Medical School, he recently established a nonprofit organization, the National Integrative Medicine Council, to advance the cause of integrative medicine through public policy, education, and research. He is the author of eight books including *Spontaneous Healing, Eight Weeks to Optimum Health,* and *Eating Well for Optimum Health*.

T E X T   A C K N O W L E D G M E N T S

Every effort has been made to trace all copyright holders of the material included in this volume, whether companies or individuals. Any omission is unintentional and we will be pleased to correct any errors in future editions of this book.

Becoming Medically Intuitive, from *Anatomy of the Spirit,* published by Harmony Books, © 1996 by Caroline Myss, used by kind permission of the author

Cancer Becomes Me, © 1997 by Marjory Gross, first published in *Surviving Crisis* edited by Lee Gutkind (Tarcher Putnam)

Cupid's Disease, © 1985 by Oliver Sacks, used by kind permission of The Wylie Agency, Inc.

De-Stress or Distress, © 2000 by Madeleine Begun Kane @ MadKane.com, used by kind permission of the author

Doctor, Talk to Me by Anatole Broyard, © 1990 by The New York Times Company, used by kind permission of *The New York Times*

Energy Medicine, from *Energy Medicine* by Donna Eden with David Feinstein, © 1998 by Donna Eden, used by kind permission of the author

Fat, ©1997 by Carol Kloss, used by kind permission of the author

Final Lesson, from *Kitchen Table Wisdom* by Rachel Naomi Remen, M.D., © 1996 by Rachel Naomi Remen, used by kind permission of Riverhead Books, a division of Penguin Putnam, Inc.

Healing and the Mind, from *Healing and the Mind* by Bill Moyers, © 1993 by Public Affairs Television and David Grubin Productions, Inc. Used by kind permission of Doubleday, a division of Random House, Inc.

Heart Attack, ©1976 by Max Apple, used by kind permission of author

Helping Patients Decide to Die, from *Denial of the Soul* by M. Scott Peck, © 1997 by M. Scott Peck. Used by kind permission of Harmony Books, a division of Random House, Inc.

House Calls, from *The Youngest Science: Notes of a Medicine Watcher* by Lewis Thomas, © 1983 by Lewis Thomas.Used by kind permission of Viking Penguin, a division of Penguin Putnam, Inc.

I Accept All the Parts of Myself, from *Heart Thoughts* by Louise L. Hay, © 1990 by Louise L. Hay. Used by permission of Hay House, Inc.

The Leaf Shape Remains, © 2000 by John Fox, used by kind permission of the author

Listening to Prozac, from *Listening to Prozac* by Peter D. Kramer, ©1993 by Peter D. Kramer. Used by kind permission of Viking Penguin, a division of Penguin Putnam, Inc.

Still Here, from *Still Here* by Ram Dass, © 2000 by Ram Dass. Used by kind permission of Riverhead Books, a division of Penguin Putnam, Inc.

Thank You M'am, from *Short Stories* by Langston Hughes, © 1996 by Ramona Bass and Arnold Rampersad. Used by kind permission of Hill and Wang, a division of Farrar, Straus and Giroux, LLC, and Harold Ober Associates Incorporated

Touching, © 2001 by David Hellerstein (www.hellerstein.net). Used by kind permission of the author

The Use of Force, from *Doctor Stories,* © 1938 by William Carlos Williams. Used by kind permission of New Directions Publishing Corporation and Laurence Pollinger Limited

What I Know from Noses, © 2000 by Andee Hochman, used by kind permission of the author

Wisteria, originally published in *Between the Heartbeats,* edited by Cortney Davis and Judy Schaefer, © 1995 by Leslie Nyman. Used by kind permission of the author

A R T   A C K N O W L E D G M E N T S

Page 9   Arthur Dove, American, 1880-1946, *Nature Symbolized No. 2,* 1911-14, pastel on paper, sheet: 45.8 x 55 cm, gift of Georgia O'Keeffe to the Alfred Stieglitz Collection, 1949.533, photo reproduction © The Art Institute of Chicago. All Rights Reserved

Page 15   Marsden Hartley, American, 1877-1943, *Movements,* c. 1915, oil on canvas, 119.7 x 120 cm, Alfred Stieglitz Collection, 1949.544, photo reproduction © The Art Institute of Chicago. All Rights Reserved

Page 16   Georgia O'Keeffe, American, 1887-1986. *It was Yellow and Pink IIII,* 1960, oil on canvas, 101.6 x 76.2cm, Alfred Stieglitz Collection, bequest of Georgia O'Keeffe, 1987.250.2, photo reproduction © The Art Institute of Chicago. All Rights Reserved

Page 18   Jacob Lawrence, American, 1917-2000, *Free Clinic,* 1937, gouache, on tan wove paper, laid down on ivory cardboard, image: 73.1 x 77.9 cm; sheet: 76.7 x 81.8 cm, H. Karl and Nancy von Maltitz Endowment, 1990.447, photo reproduction © The Art Institute of Chicago. All Rights Reserved

Page 25   Courtesy of *The Advertising Archives*

Page 29   Grandma Moses, American, 1860-1961, *Making Apple Butter,* 1958, oil on panel, 12 x 16 in, Gift of Mrs. Ignatius Jelinski, 1976.428. Reproduction © The Art Institute of Chicago. All Rights Reserved

Page 30   Getty Images/Hulton Archive

Page 34   Georgia O'Keeffe, American, 1887-1986. *Abstraction – White Rose III,* 1927, oil on canvas, 91.4 x 76.2 cm, Alfred Stieglitz Collection, bequest of Georgia O'Keeffe, 1987.250.1, photo reproduction © The Art Institute of Chicago. All Rights Reserved

Page 38   Agnes Pelton, *Lotus for Lida.* Private collection, courtesy of Kelley Gallery, Pasadena, California

Page 41   Charles Burchfield, *Woodpecker;* Reynolda House, Museum of American Art, Winston-Salem, North Carolina. Reproduction rights courtesy of The Charles E. Burchfield Foundation and Kennedy Galleries, Inc., New York

Page 42   Agnes Pelton, *Sea Change,* 1931, oil on canvas, 20 x 28 3/16 in. (50.8 x 71.6 cm). Whitney Museum of American Art, New York; gift of Lois and Irvin Cohen, 99.64

Page 43   Mary Evans Picture Library

Page 48   Julie Foakes

Page 52   John K. Hillers, *Navaho Shaman, ca. 1886,* albumen silver print, P1967.2552, Amon Carter Museum, Fort Worth, Texas

Page 57   Eliot Porter, *Apples on Tree After Frost,* Tesuques, New Mexico, November 21, 1966, dye transfer print, P1989.19.41; © 1990, Amon Carter Museum, Fort Worth, Texas, Gift of the artist

Page 60   Gaston Lachaise, American, 1882-1935, *Standing Woman,* 1927, bronze, 185.2 x 71.1 cm, base: 43.8 x 53.3 cm, Friends of American Art Collection, 1943.580, photo reproduction © The Art Institute of Chicago. All Rights Reserved

Page 64   Giles Horton, *Anaesthetic or not*

Page 69   Alfred Stieglitz, American 1864-1946, *Georgia O'Keeffe,* 1920, platinum print, 25.3 x 20.3 cm, The Alfred Stieglitz Collection, 1949.756, photo reproduction © The Art Institute of Chicago. All Rights Reserved

Page 70   Sarah Pletts, *Elements,* 1993, photomontage, 18" x 12"

Page 113   Georgia O'Keeffe, American, 1887-1986. *Blue and Green Music,* 1919, oil on canvas, 8.4 x 48.3 cm, Alfred Stieglitz Collection, gift of Georgia O'Keeffe, 1969.835, photo reproduction © The Art Institute of Chicago. All Rights Reserved

Page 119   Sarah Pletts, *Warped Fruit III,* 1994, digital image

Page 120   Lucas Samaras, *Skull & Milky Way,* 1966. X-ray photograph and pins, 29 1/4 x 25 3/8 x 3 3/4 in. (73.34 x 62.87 x 8.89 cm.), Whitney Museum of American Art, New York; gift of Howard and Jean Lipman, 91.34.6. © Lucas Samaras

Page 121   Sarah Pletts, *Intensive Care,* 1988, charcoal on paper, 838 x 1143 mm

Page 125   Georgia O'Keeffe, American, 1887-1986. *Black Rock with Blue Sky and White Clouds,* 1972, oil on canvas, 91.4 x 76.8 cm, Alfred Stieglitz Collection, bequest of Georgia O'Keeffe, 1987.250.3, photo reproduction © The Art Institute of Chicago. All Rights Reserved

Page 126   Andrew Lane

Page 127   Nick Andrew, *Chirallo*

Page 131   Julian Onderdonk, *A Cloudy Day, Bluebonnets near San Antonio, Texas,* 1918, oil on canvas, 1998.10; Amon Carter Museum, Fort Worth, Texas, Purchase with funds from the Ruth Carter Stevenson Acquisition endowment in honor of Lady Bird Johnson

Cover   Willem de Kooning, 1939, *Seated Figure (Classic Male),* oil on plywood, 138 x 91.5 cm, Daros Collection, Switzerland. © 2002 The Willem de Kooning Foundation / Artists Rights Society (ARS), New York